THE
ULTIMATE
REP MAX X4
TRANSFORMATION
WORKOUTS III

The ULTIMATE REP MAX X4 TRANSFORMATION

WORKOUTS III

The Best workout routines to build muscle, increase strength, and sculpt the best body with the power of the Bullworker and the Iso-bow!

BECOME A POWERFUL!

The Ultimate Rep Max X4 Transformation Workouts III was written to help you get closer to your physical potential when it comes to real muscle sculpting strengthening exercises. The exercises and routines in this book are quite demanding, so consult your physician and have a physical exam taken prior to the start of this exercise program. Proceed with the suggested exercises and information at your own risk. The Publishers and author shall not be liable or responsible for any loss, injury, or damage allegedly arising from the information or suggestions in this book.

The Ultimate Rep Max X4 Transformation Workouts III
a muscle-building master-plan

By

Birch Tree Publishing
Published by Birch Tree Publishing

Birch Tree Publishing

Dedication

Build Powerful Muscles **TODAY!**

Contents

A Powerful Body Starts Here

BUILD YOUR BODY "GET" TRANSFORMED

with The Ultimate Rep Max X3 Transformation Workouts III the fastest muscle-producing series in the palms of your hands!

Introduction by Marlon Birch CSCS

Trainees of my Bullworker Series" know that I present the best muscle-building programs to increase optimum strength and add quality to one's life. That's my ultimate goal with my muscle enhancing programs.

This book introduces The Ultimate Rep Max X3 Transformation Workouts III these programs will get you in the best shape **FASTER** than you thought possible. With the power of our system and the muscle-building benefits of isometrics holds. Combining Isotonics and Isometrics forces the muscles to contract harder and over come neuromuscular system failure.

Our methods extend a set beyond failure, and you will see muscle popping up almost overnight. While getting more muscular and leaner than ever before. It's an eye-opening program that can help you pack on muscle and strength fast. We also look at the optimal rep speed for you to keep building muscles while applying various factors to increase growth.

Keep moving forward

Marlon Birch

Yours In Health and Strength

FULL-BODY WORKOUTS

CHAPTER 1
HYPER-MAX X2
PHASE ONE
2 WEEKS
REP SPEED CONTRACT 2 SECONDS, RELEASE 2 SECONDS

01 HYPER MAX X2 PHASE ONE

Perform 20 reps, on the 20th rep perform a 20 second Isometric contraction. All exercises are done non stop until one round is finished. Rest 5 seconds between rounds. Alternate day one and day two for 6 days per week.

DAY ONE

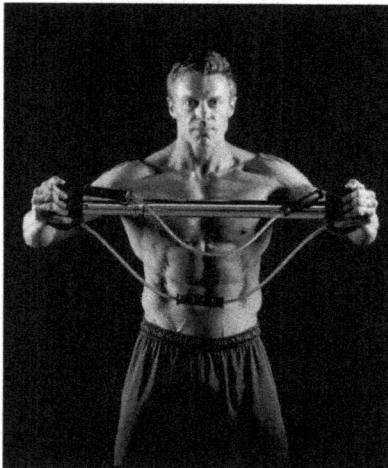
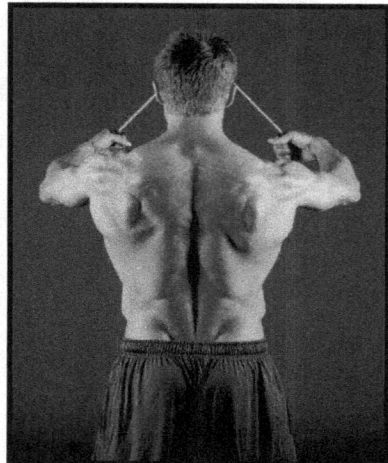
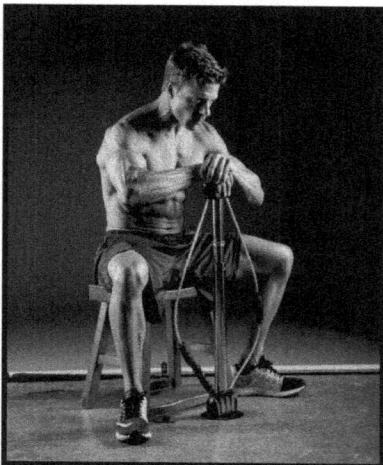
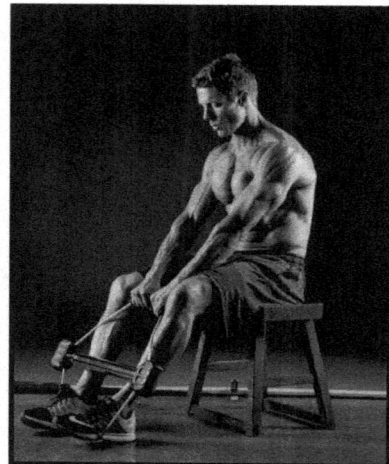

01 HYPER MAX X2 PHASE ONE

DAY ONE CONTINUED.....

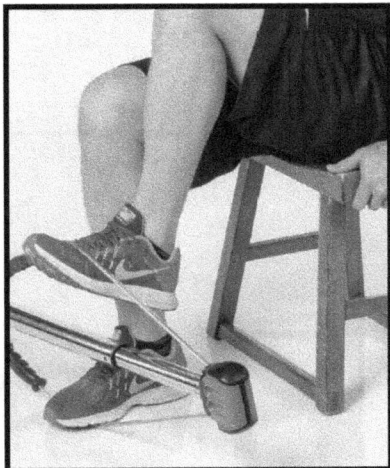

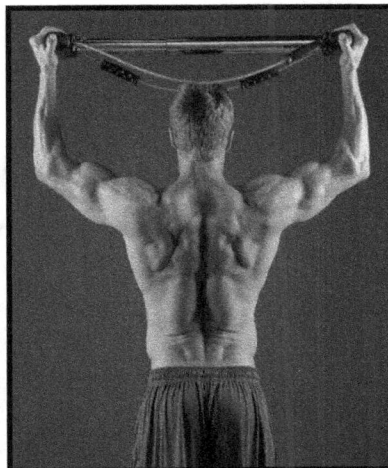

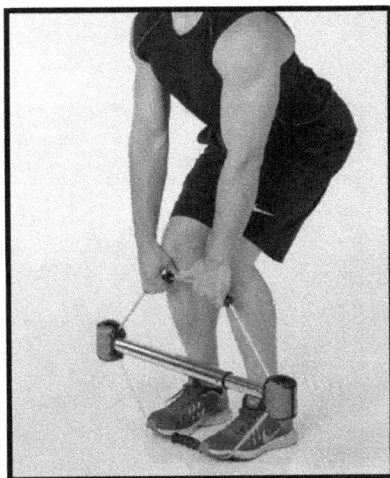

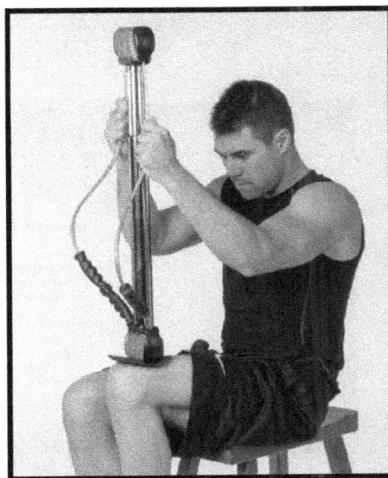

01 HYPER MAX X2

DAY TWO

Same instructions as Day one.

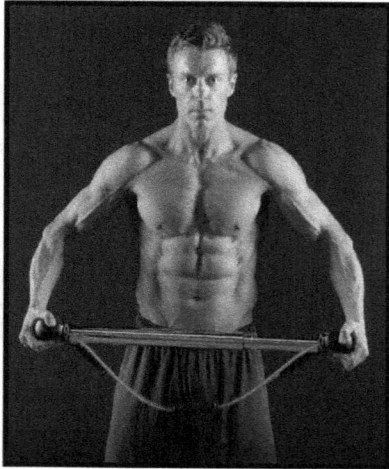

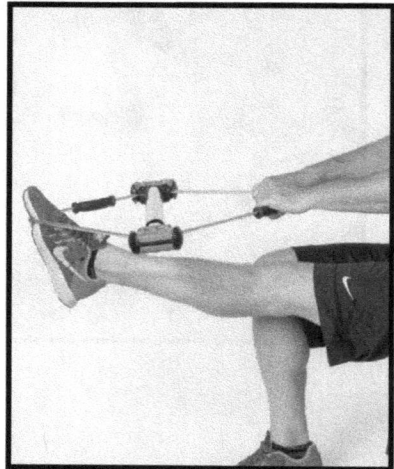

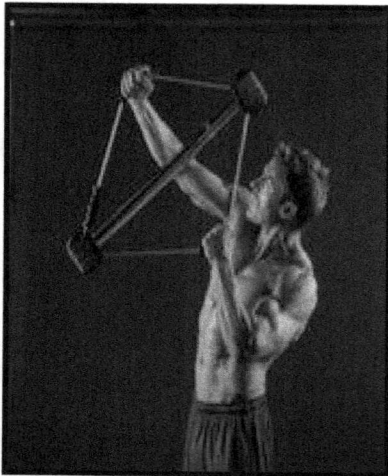

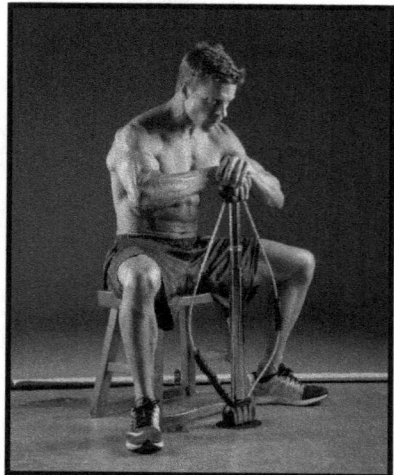

01 HYPER MAX X2
DAY TWO CONTINUED.......

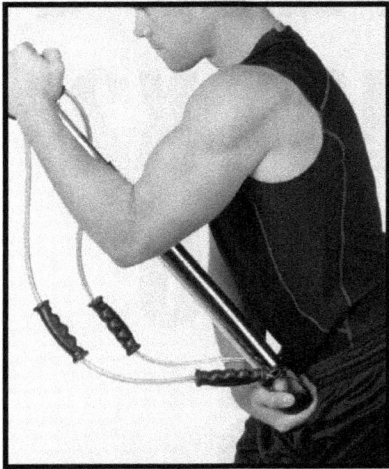

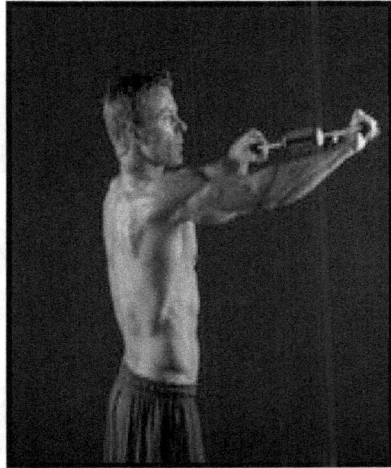

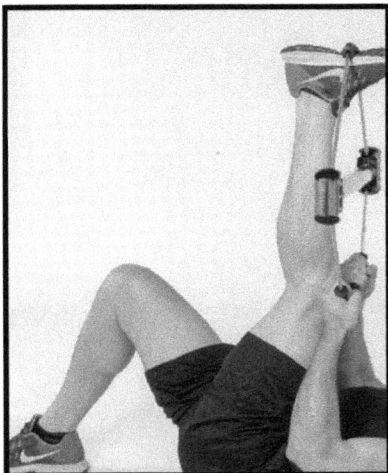

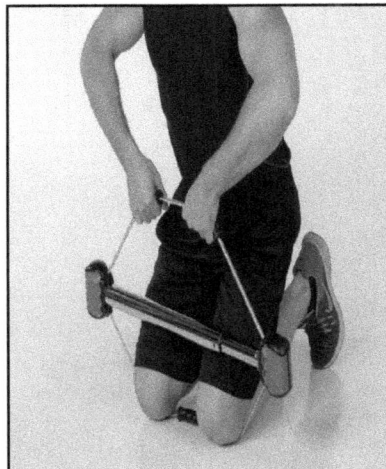

CHAPTER 1
HYPER MAX X2

PHASE TWO

3 WEEKS
REP SPEED CONTRACT 2 SECONDS, RELEASE 2 SECONDS

01 HYPER MAX X2

Perform 20 full reps, followed by 10 half reps. At the start position to the mid-point of the exercise stroke. On the 10th half rep perform a 20 second Isometric contraction. All exercises are done non stop until one round is finished. Perform 3 rounds Rest 5 seconds between rounds. Alternate day one and day two for 6 days per week.

DAY ONE

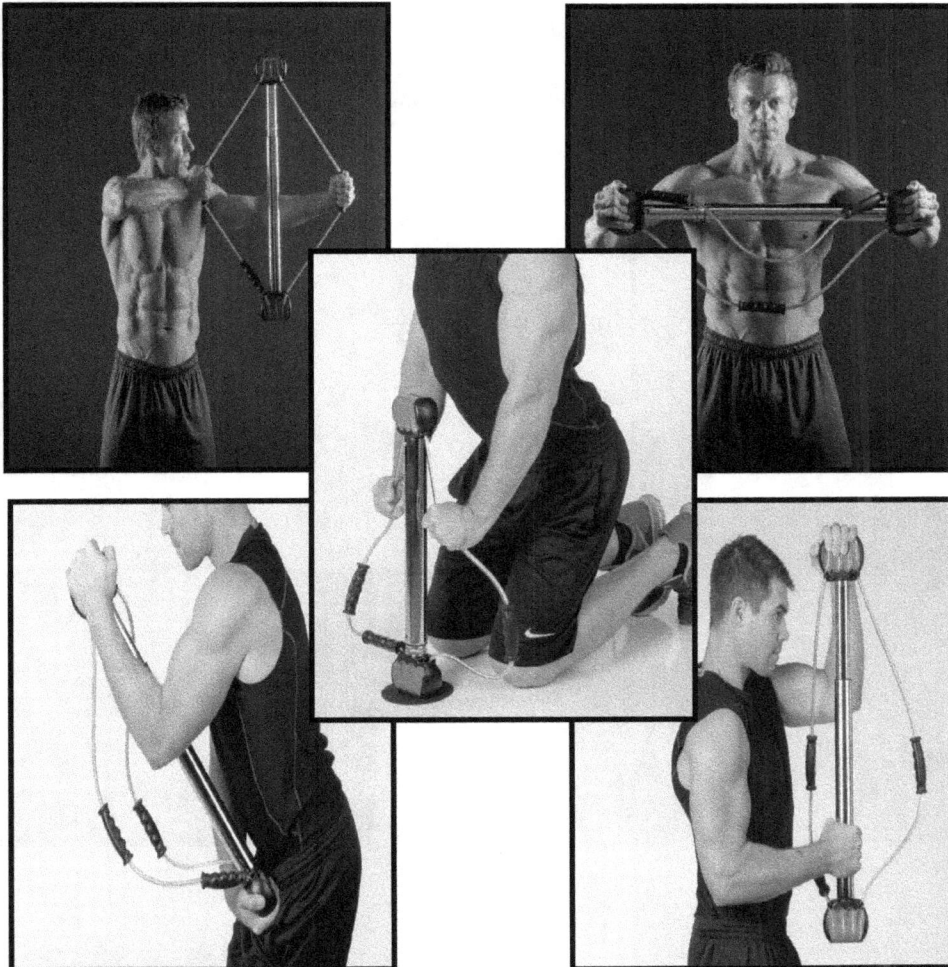

01 HYPER MAX X2

DAY TWO

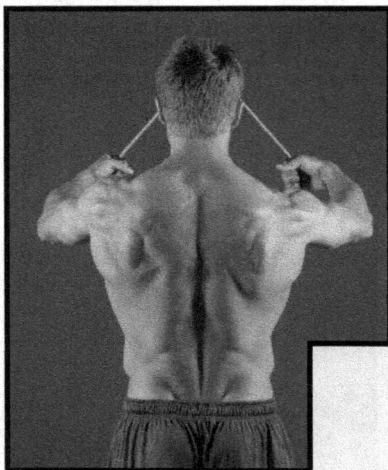
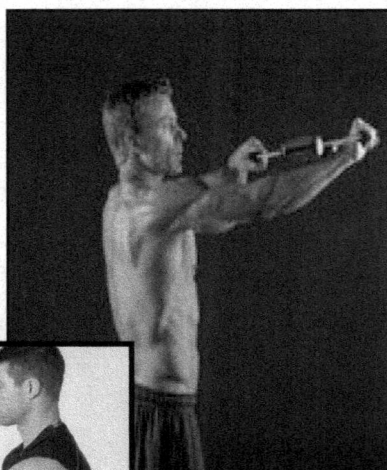
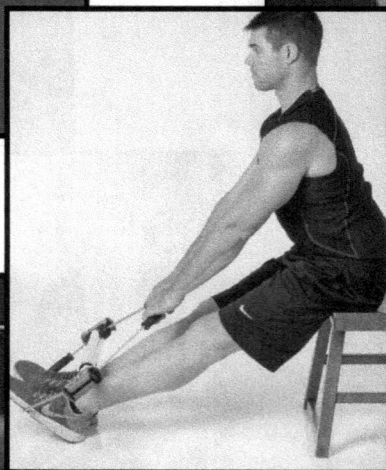
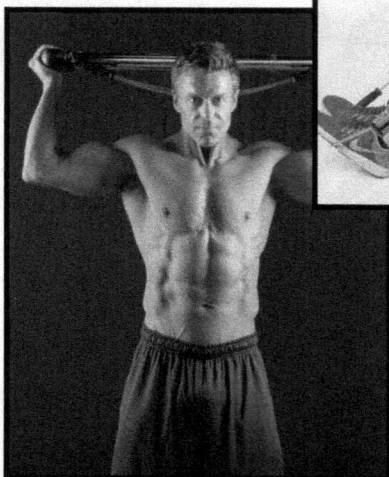
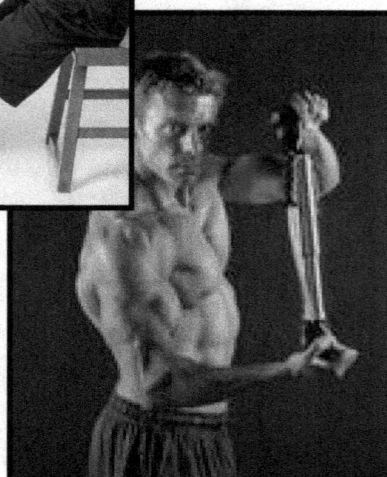

CHAPTER 2

HYPER-PUMP X2

PHASE THREE

2 WEEKS

REP SPEED CONTRACT 2 SECONDS, RELEASE 2 SECONDS

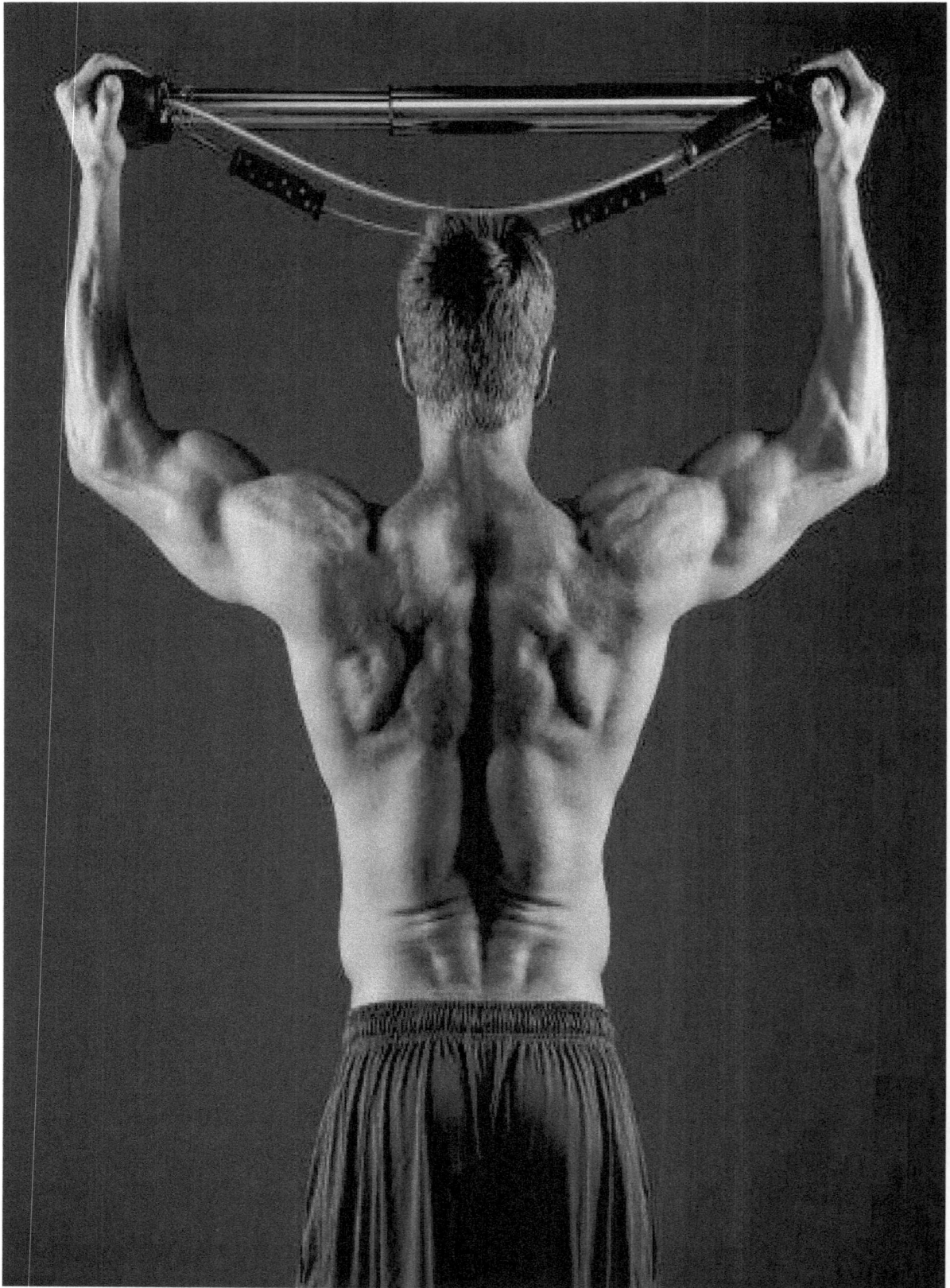

02 HYPER-PUMP X2

Perform all exercises non-stop. Perform 30 reps per exercise, on the 30th rep perform a 20 second isometric hold. Three rounds in total.

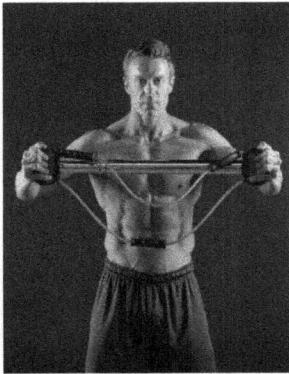
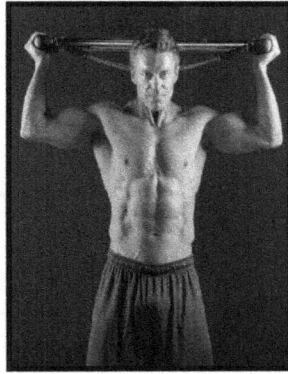
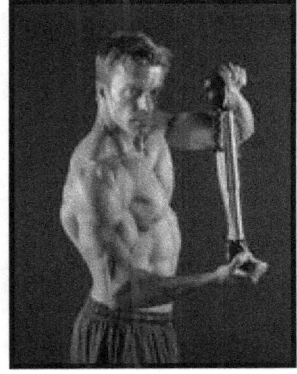

MON, WED, FRI

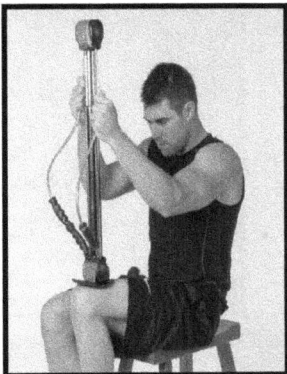
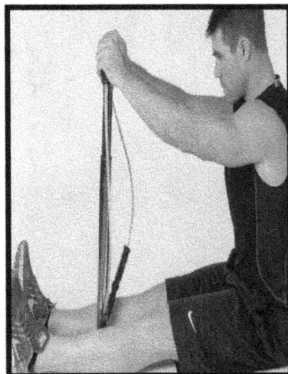
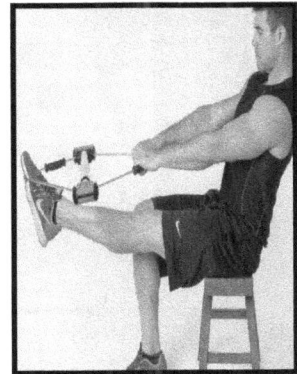

02 MAX SURGE PROGRAM

Perform all exercises non-stop. Perform 30 reps per exercise, on the 30th rep perform a 20 second isometric hold. Three rounds in total.

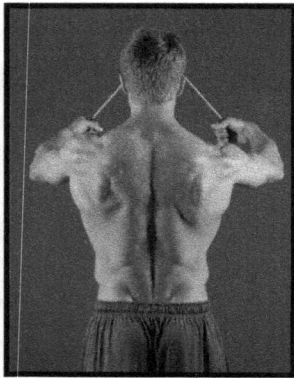

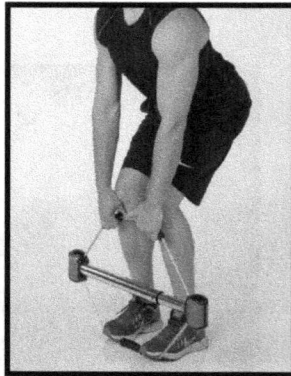

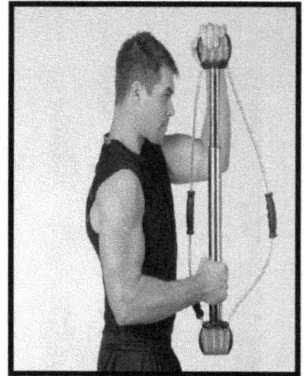

TUES, THURS, SAT

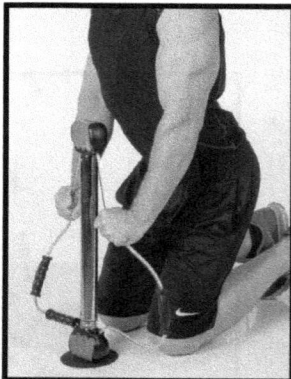

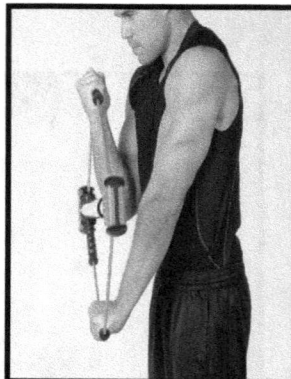

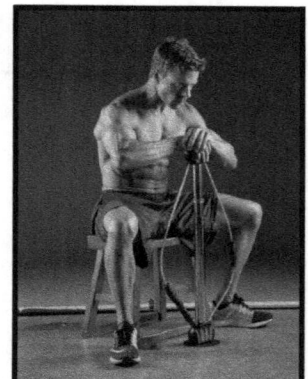

CHAPTER 2
HYPER PUMP X3
PHASE FOUR
3 WEEKS
REP SPEED CONTRACT 2 SECONDS, RELEASE 2 SECONDS

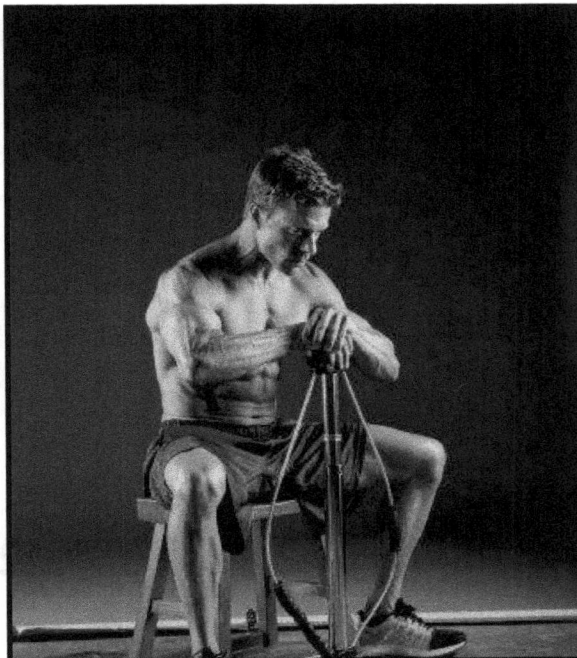

02 HYPER PUMP X3

Perform 30 reps, on the 30th rep perform a 30 second Isometric contraction. All exercises are done non stop until one round is finished. Perform two rounds, rest 5 seconds between rounds.

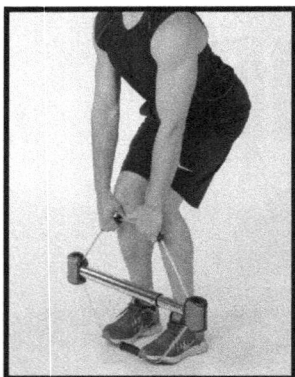
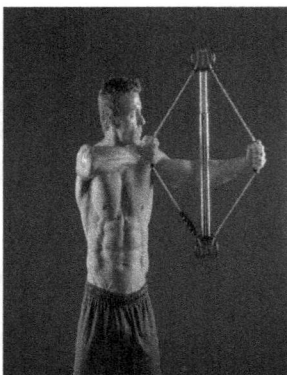
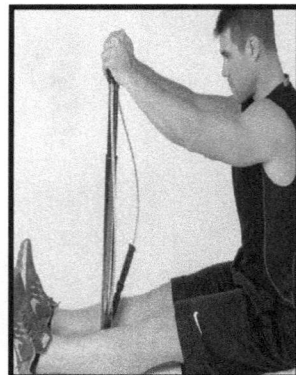

MON, WED, FRI

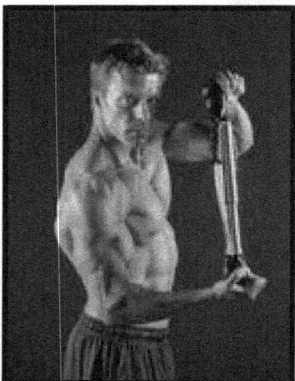
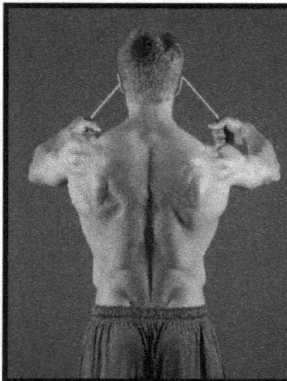
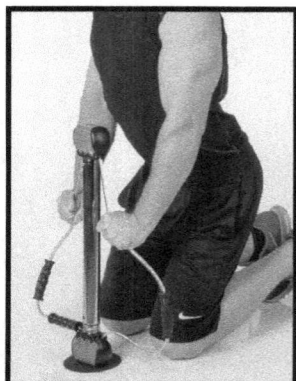

02 HYPER PUMP X3

Perform 30 reps, on the 30th rep perform a 30 second Isometric contraction. All exercises are done non stop until one round is finished. Perform two rounds, rest 5 seconds between rounds.

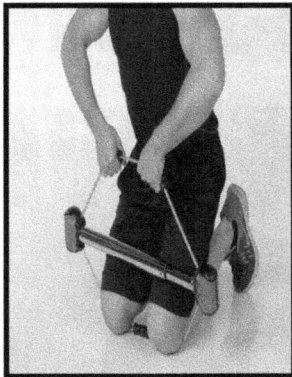

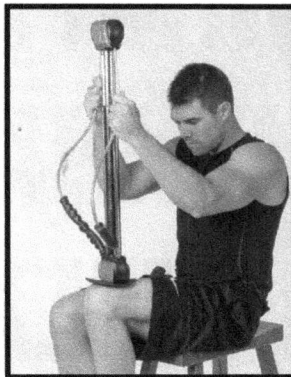

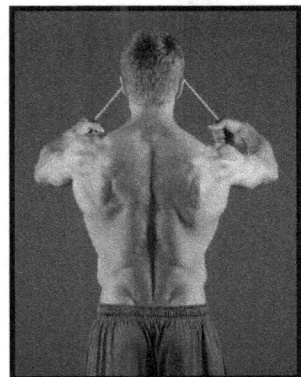

TUES, THURS, SAT

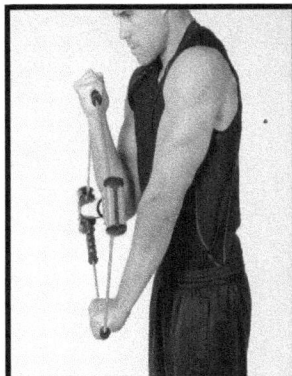

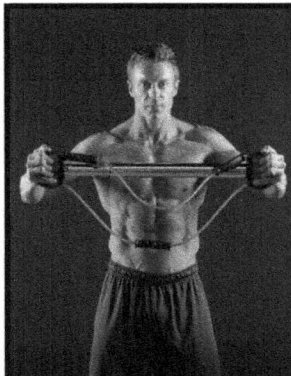

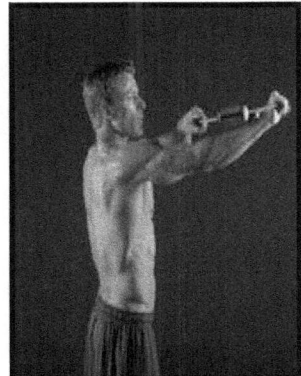

CHAPTER 3
SUPERCOMPENSATION
MAX X5 PHASE FIVE
3 WEEKS
REP SPEED CONTRACT 2 SECONDS, RELEASE 2 SECONDS

03 MAX 5 PROGRAM

Perform a 20 second Isometric contraction, followed by 5 reps. On the 5th rep perform another 20 second contraction. Perform all exercises non-stop until one full round is completed. Rest 5 seconds and complete 3 rounds.

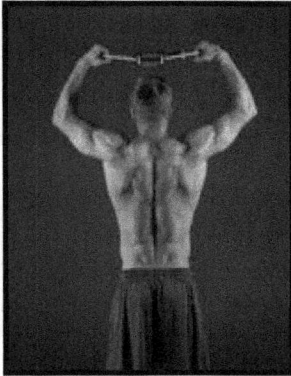
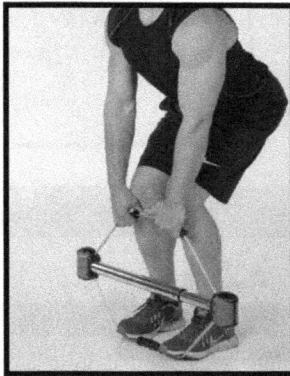
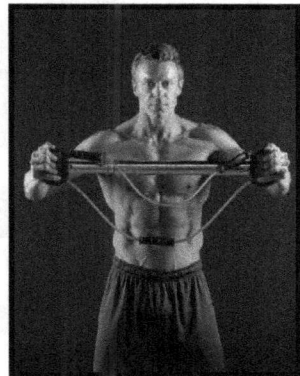

MON, WED, FRI

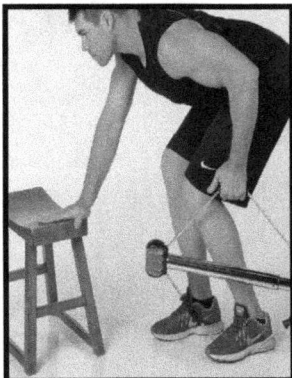
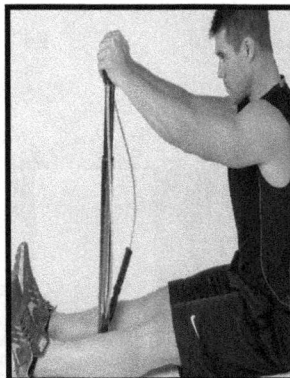
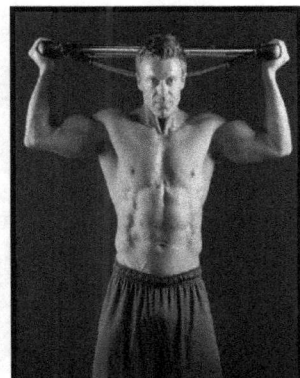

03 MAX 5 PROGRAM

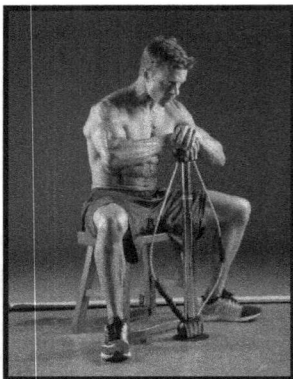

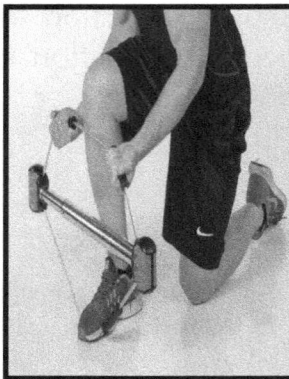

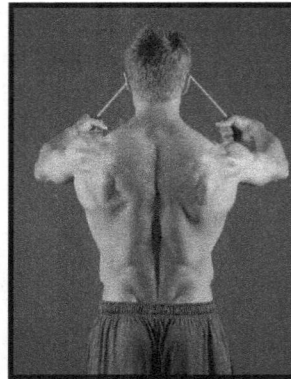

TUES, THURS, SAT

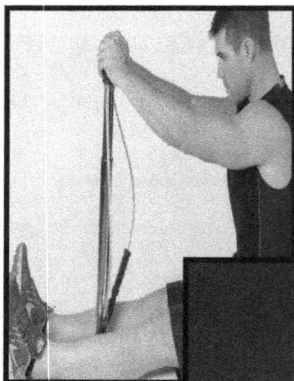

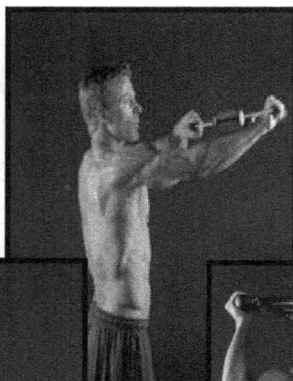

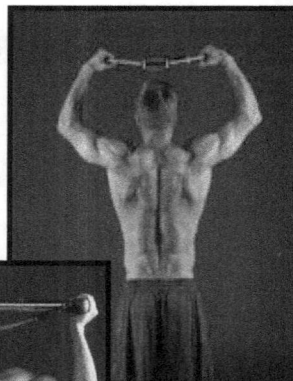

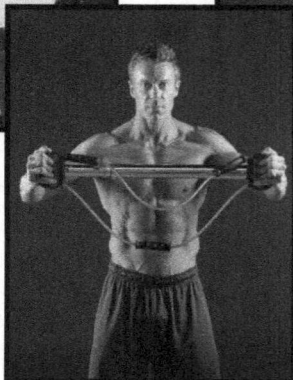

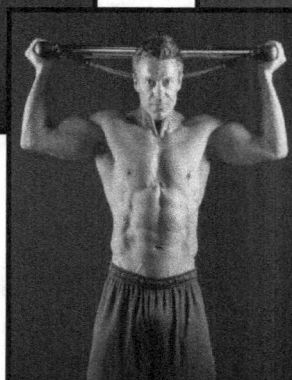

CHAPTER 3
SUPERCOMPENSATION
MAX X5 PHASE SIX
2 WEEKS
REP SPEED CONTRACT 2 SECONDS, RELEASE 2 SECONDS

03 MAX X5 PROGRAM

Perform a 20 second Isometric contraction, followed by 10 reps. On the 10th rep perform another 20 second isometric contraction. Perform all exercises non-stop until one full round is completed. Rest 5 seconds and complete 3 rounds.

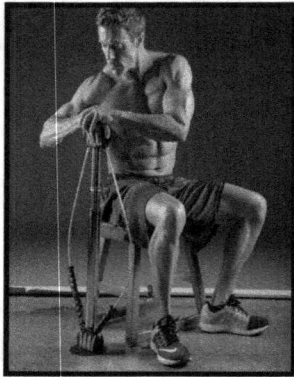 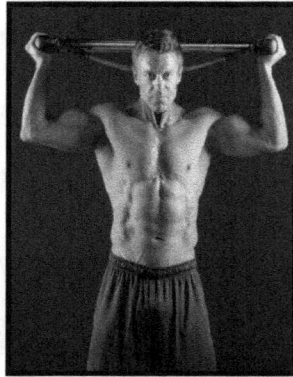 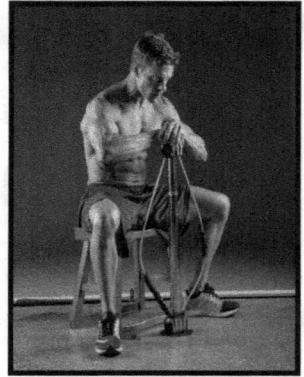

MON, WED, FRI

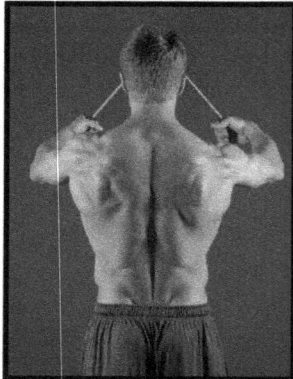 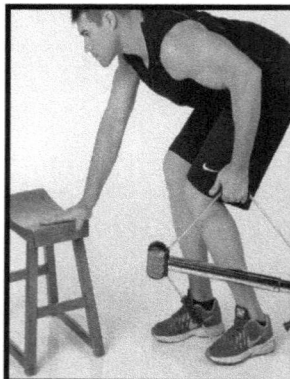 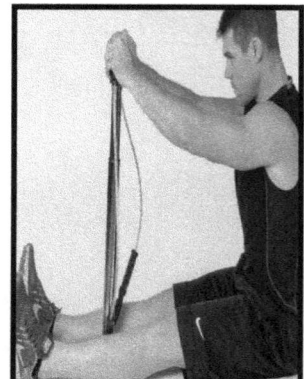

03 MAX X5 PROGRAM

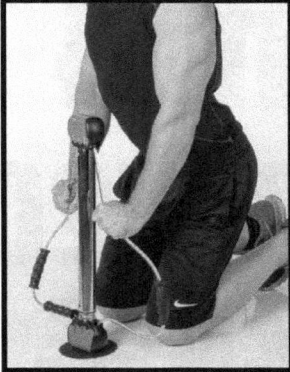

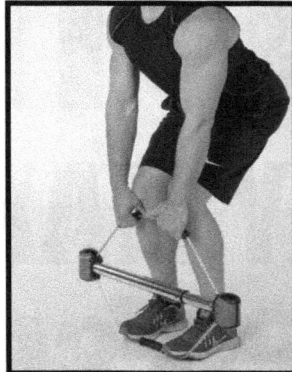

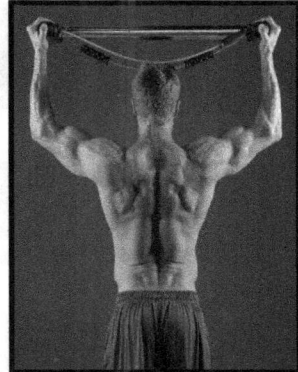

TUES, THURS, SAT

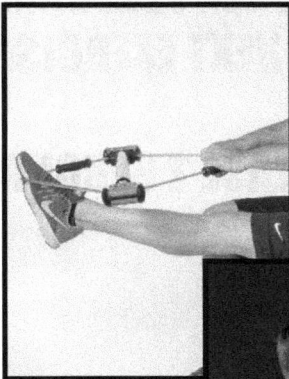

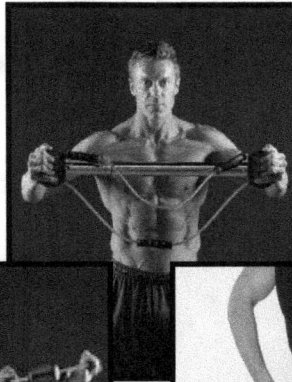

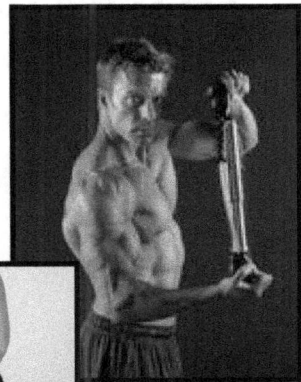

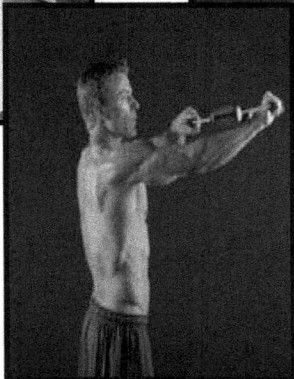

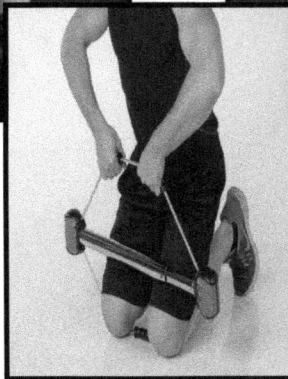

CHAPTER 4
DENSITY MAX 20X20
PHASE SEVEN
3 WEEKS

PERFORM 20 REPS, REST 5 SECONDS THEN PERFORM ANOTHER 20 REPS THEN MOVE TO THE NEXT EXERCISE

REP SPEED CONTRACT 2 SECONDS, RELEASE 2 SECONDS

04 DENSITY MAX 20X20

On each exercise perform 20x20 reps. At the end of each 20 perform a 10 second isometric contraction. Continue until all bodyparts are completed. Perform 3 rounds in total.

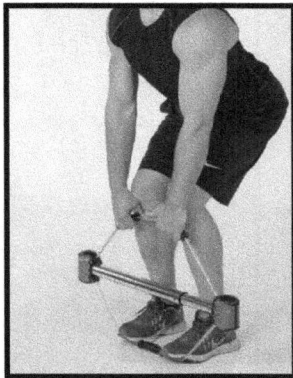
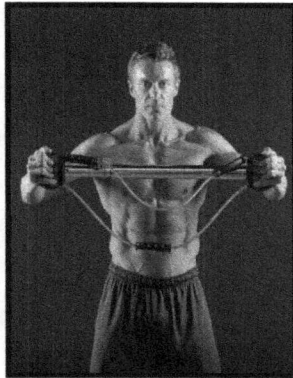
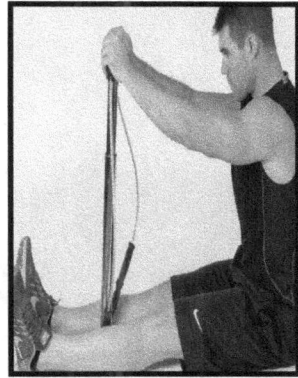

MON, WED, FRI

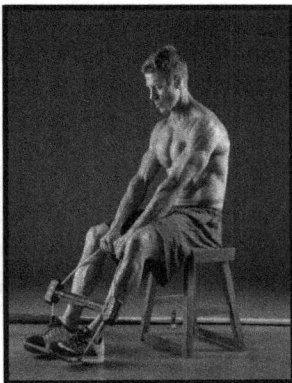
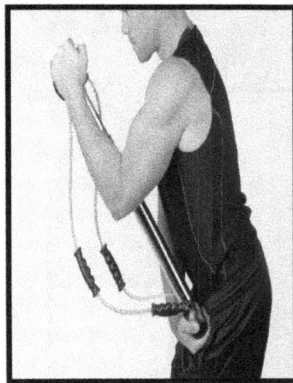
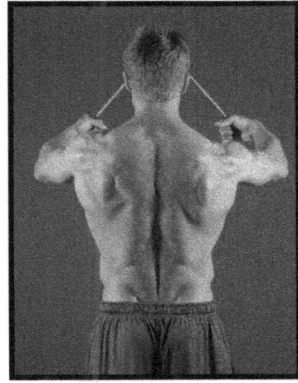

04 DENSITY MAX 20X20

On each exercise perform 20x20 reps. At the end of each 20 perform a 10 second isometric contraction. Continue until all bodyparts are completed. Perform 3 rounds in total.

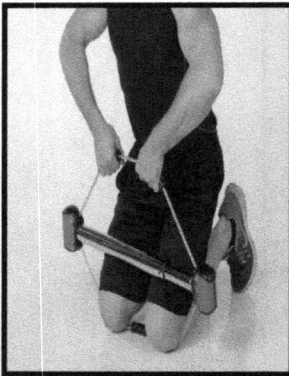

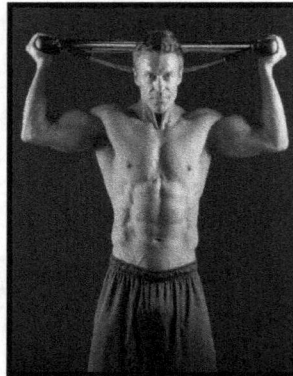

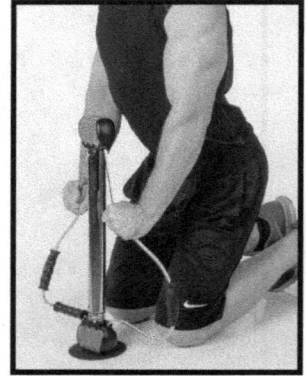

TUES, THURS, SAT

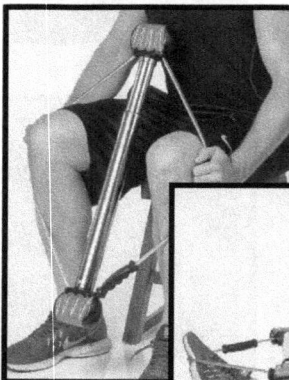

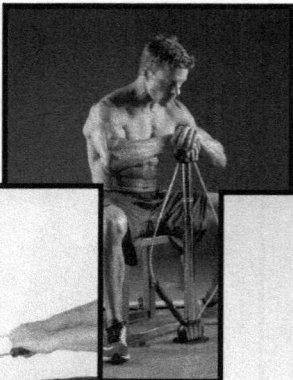

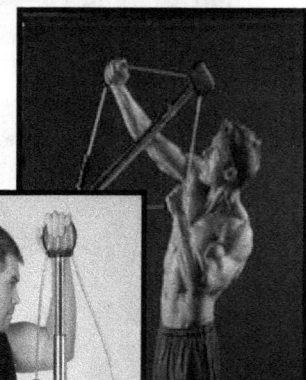

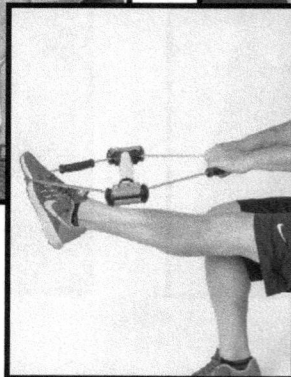

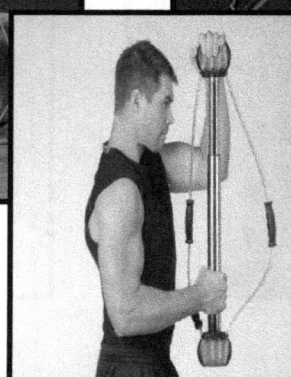

CHAPTER 5
HYPO 90 METHOD
PHASE EIGHT
3 WEEKS
REP SPEED CONTRACT 2 SECONDS, RELEASE 2 SECONDS

HYPO 90 METHOD

05 HYPO 90 METHOD DAY ONE

HOW TO PERFORM THIS ROUTINE: Perform 10 reps, followed by a 20 second isometric contraction. **PERFORM 3 ROUNDS (SETS)**

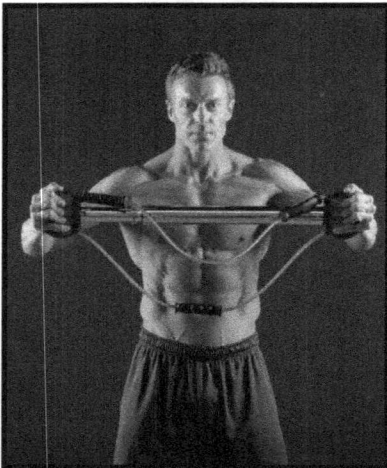

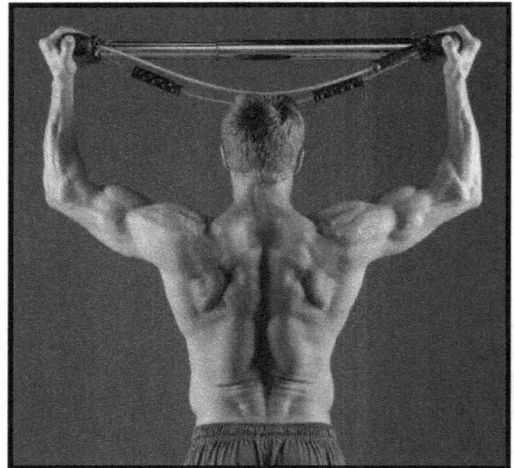

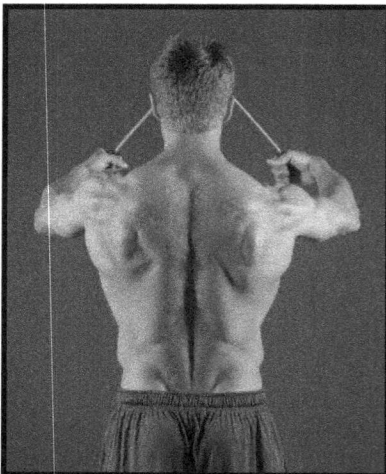

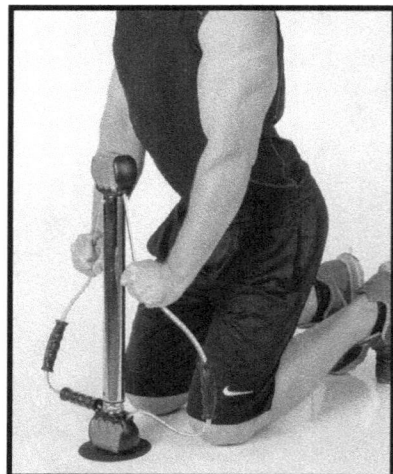

HYPO 90 METHOD

05 HYPO 90 METHOD DAY TWO

HOW TO PERFORM THIS ROUTINE: Perform 10 reps, followed by a 20 second isometric contraction. **PERFORM 3 ROUNDS (SETS)**

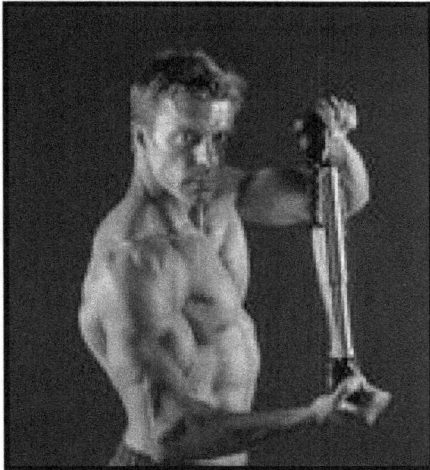
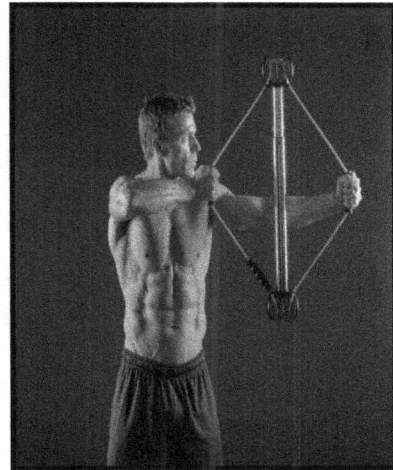
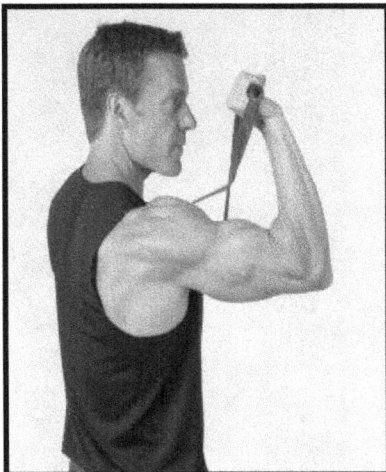
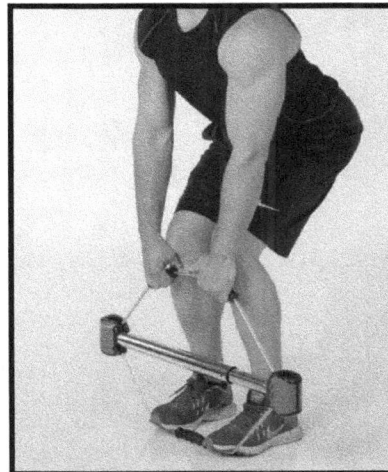

HYPO 90 METHOD

05 HYPO 90 METHOD DAY THREE

HOW TO PERFORM THIS ROUTINE: Perform 10 reps, followed by a 20 second isometric contraction. **PERFORM 3 ROUNDS (SETS)**

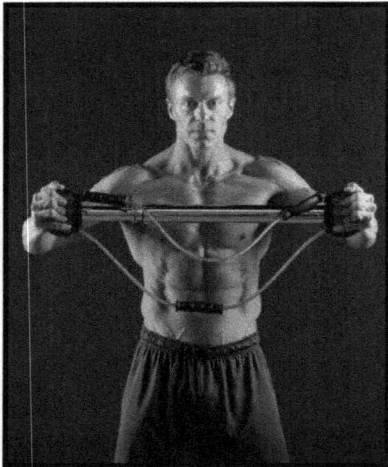

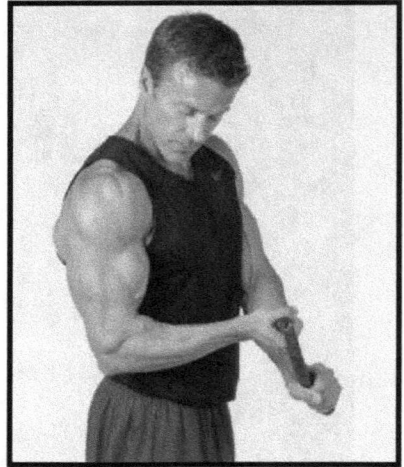

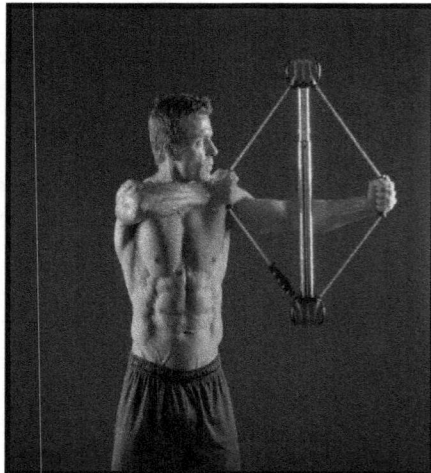

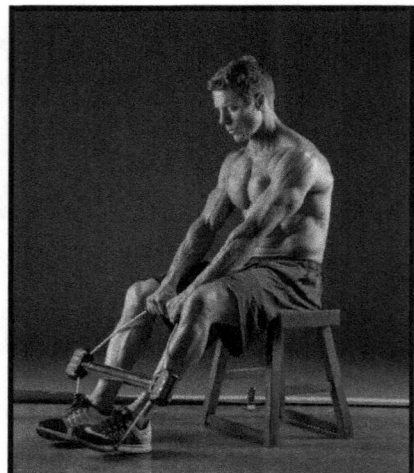

HYPO 90 METHOD

05 HYPO 90 METHOD DAY FOUR

HOW TO PERFORM THIS ROUTINE: Perform 10 reps, followed by a 20 second isometric contraction. **PERFORM 3 ROUNDS (SETS)**

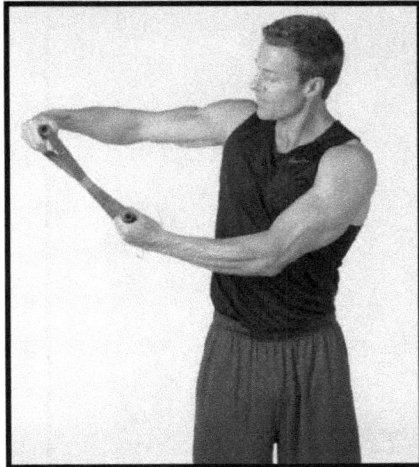
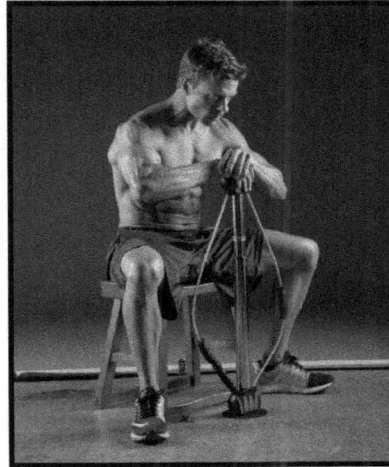
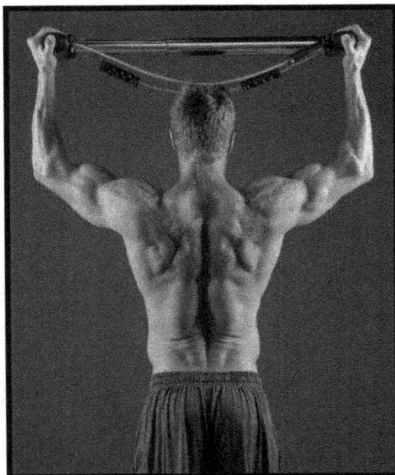
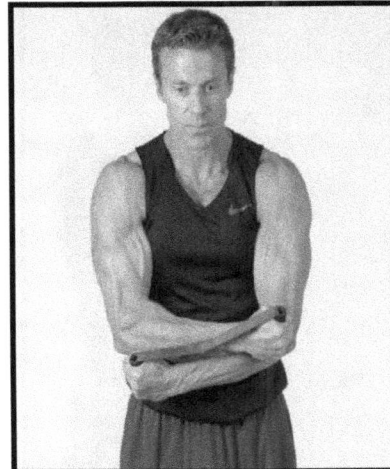

HYPO 90 METHOD

05 HYPO 90 METHOD DAY FIVE

HOW TO PERFORM THIS ROUTINE: Perform 10 reps, followed by a 20 second isometric contraction. **PERFORM 3 ROUNDS (SETS)**

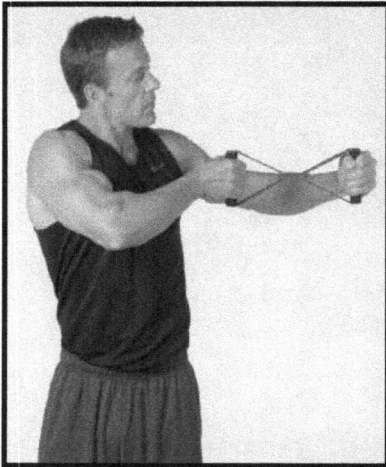

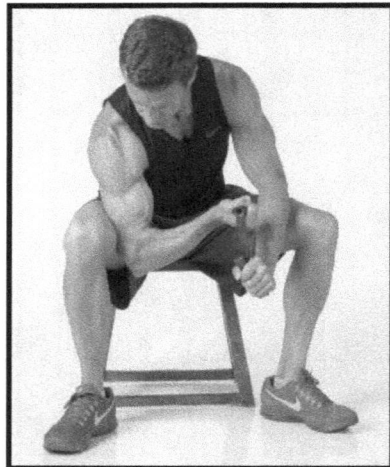

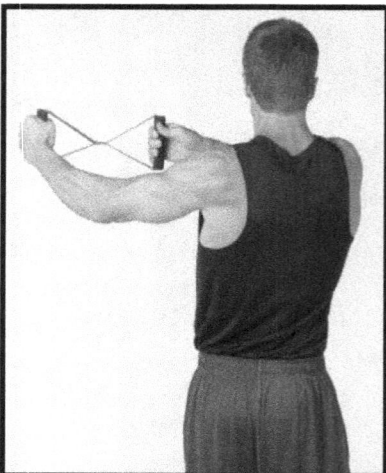

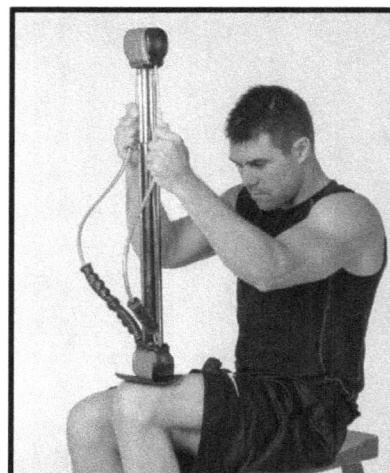

PHASE NINE

06 POWER X-FRAME METHOD

MONDAY, WEDNESDAY, FRIDAY
HOW TO PERFORM THIS ROUTINE: You contract for 2 seconds and release for a slow 10 seconds. On the last rep perform an isometric contraction for 20 seconds. Perform 2 rounds. Perform all exercises rest 10 seconds and repeat. **Perform plan for 3 weeks before moving to Phase Ten.**

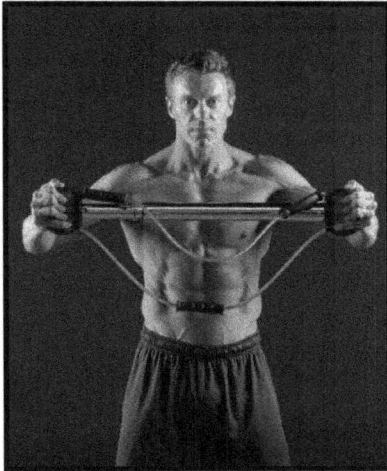

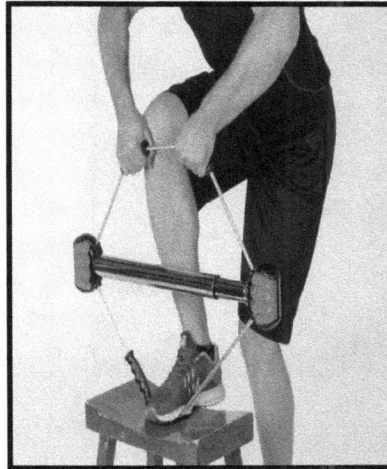

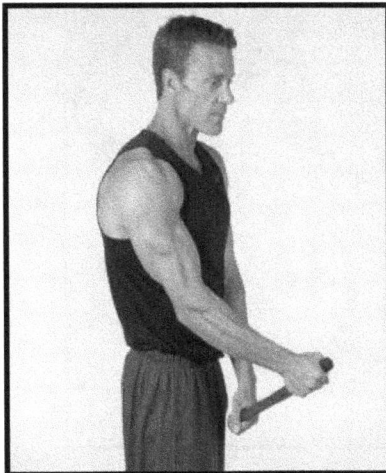

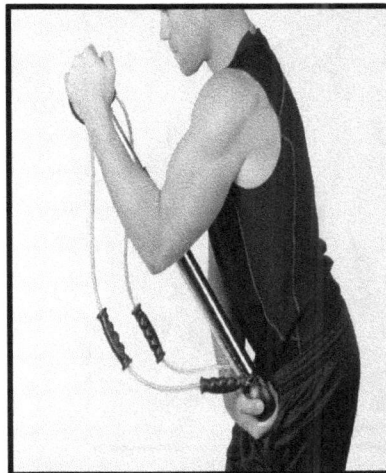

PHASE NINE

06 POWER X-FRAME METHOD

MONDAY,WEDNESDAY,FRIDAY
Routine continued.............

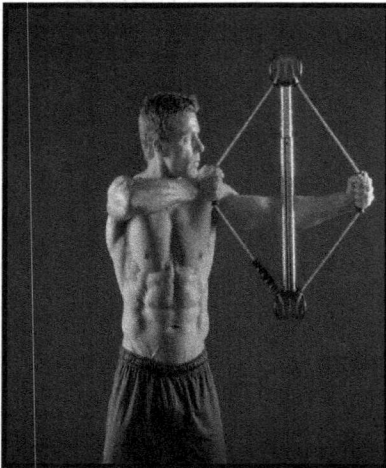

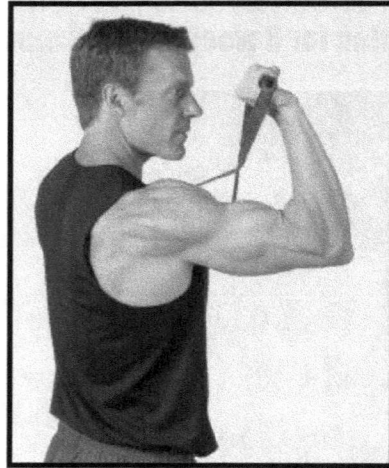

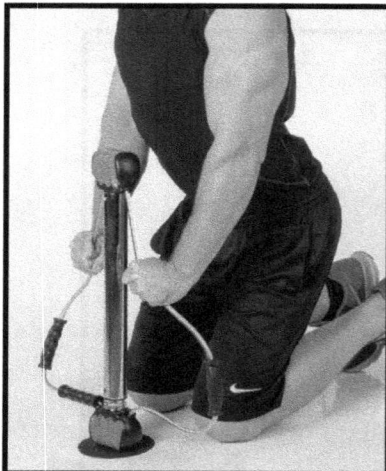

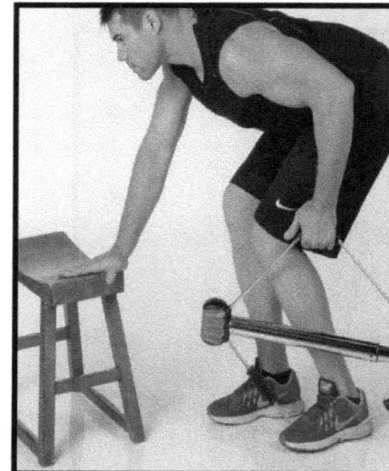

PHASE NINE

06 POWER X-FRAME METHOD

MONDAY, WEDNESDAY, FRIDAY
Routine continued............

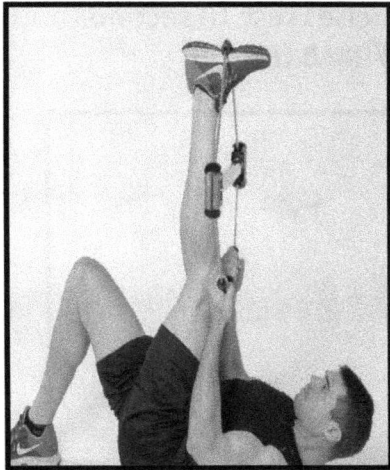

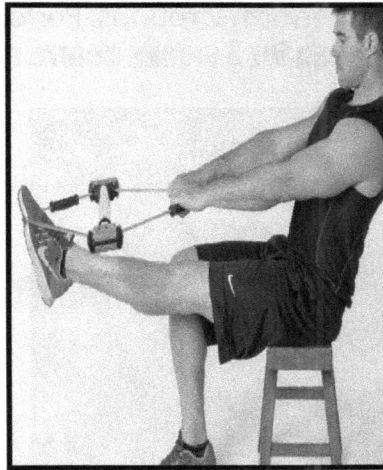

PHASE NINE MON, WED, FRI

PHASE NINE

06 POWER X-FRAME METHOD

TUESDAY, THURSDAY, SATURDAY
HOW TO PERFORM THIS ROUTINE: You contract for 2 seconds and release for a slow 10 seconds. On the last rep perform an isometric contraction for 20 seconds. Perform 2 rounds. Perform all exercises rest 10 seconds and repeat. **Perform plan for 3 weeks before moving to Phase Ten.**

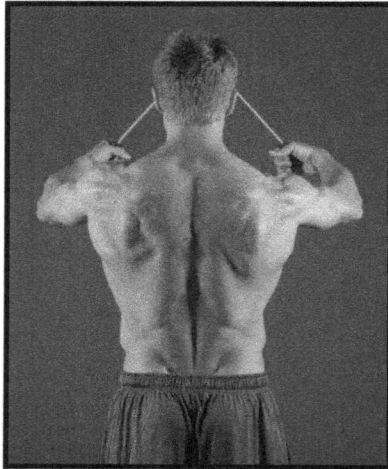

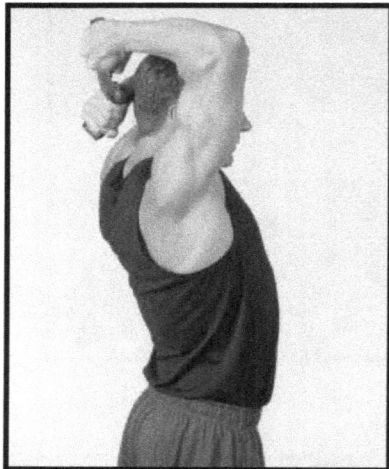

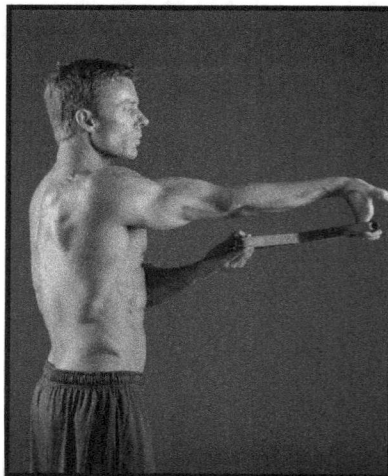

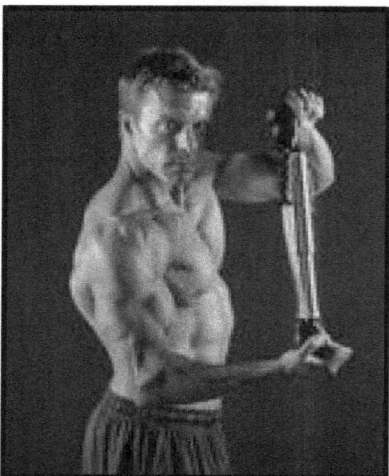

PHASE NINE

06 POWER X-FRAME METHOD

TUESDAY, THURSDAY, SATURDAY
Routine continued...................

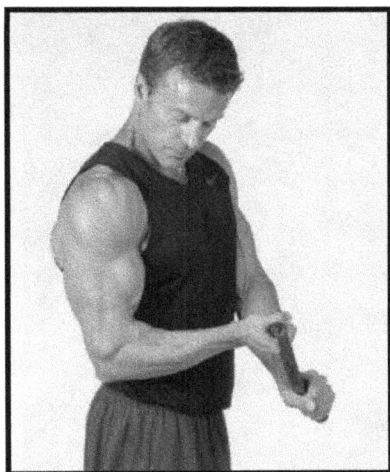

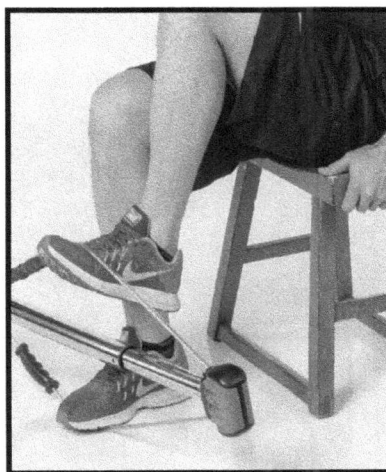

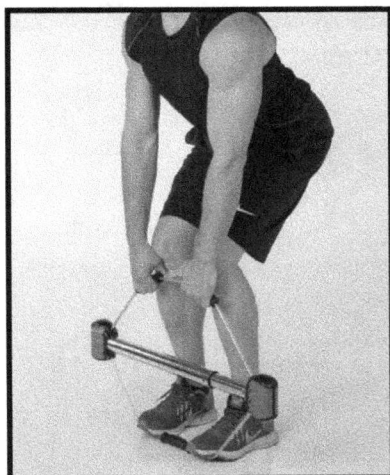

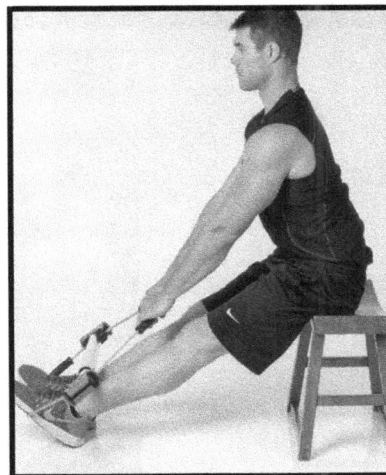

PHASE NINE

06 POWER X-FRAME METHOD

TUESDAY, THURSDAY, SATURDAY
Routine continued...................

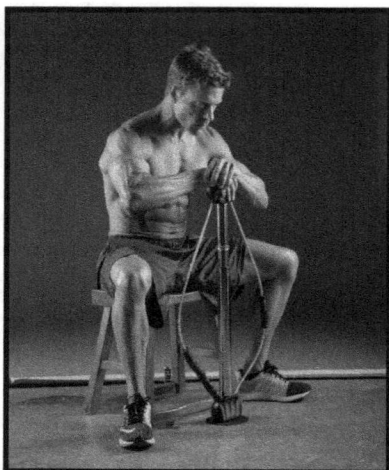

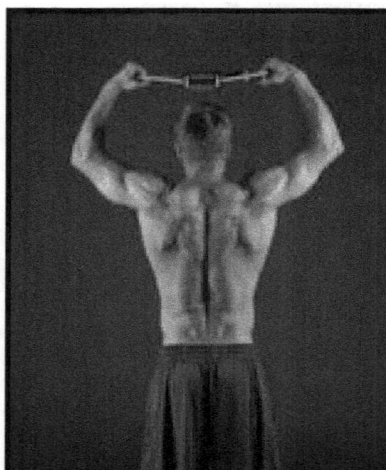

PHASE NINE TUES, THURS, SAT.

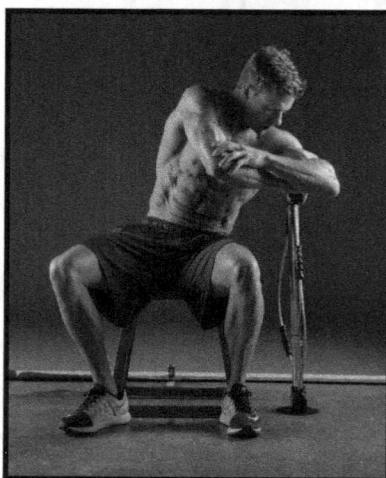

PHASE TEN

07 HYPER-DENSITY X3 METHOD 10,10,7

MONDAY, WEDNESDAY, FRIDAY
HOW TO PERFORM THIS ROUTINE: Contract 2 seconds release 2 seconds. Perform 10 reps followed by a 1 second isometric, 10 reps followed by another 1 second isometric, then a final 7 reps. On the 7th rep hold for a 10 second Isometric contraction. Perform 2 rounds. **Perform program for 3 weeks**

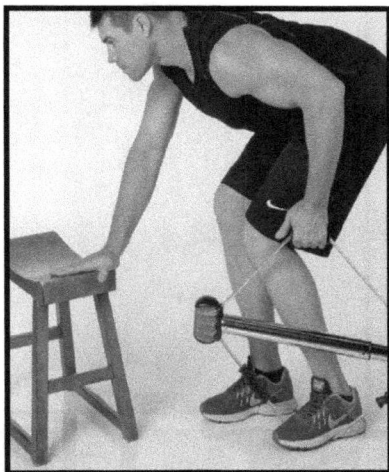

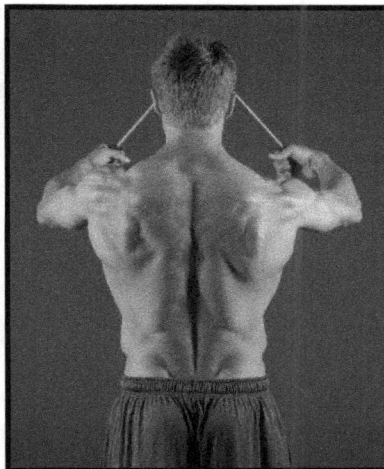

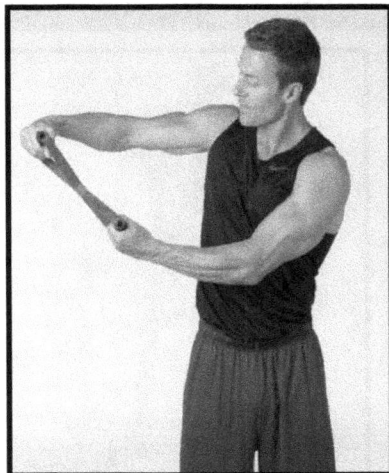

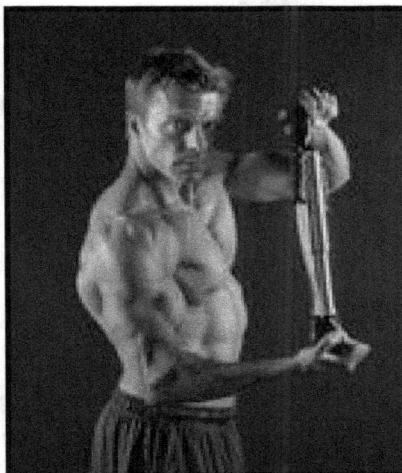

PHASE TEN

07 HYPER-DENSITY X3 METHOD 10,10,7

MONDAY, WEDNESDAY, FRIDAY
Routine continued............

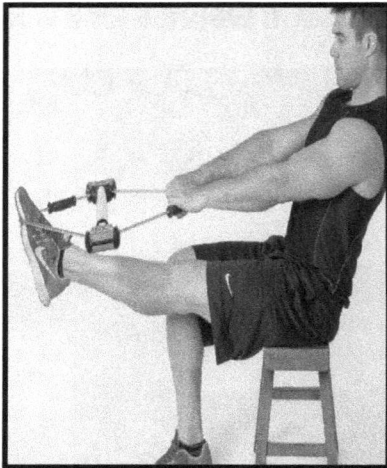

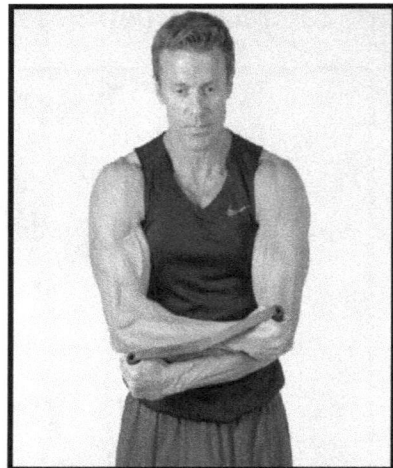

PHASE TEN   MON, WED, FRI.

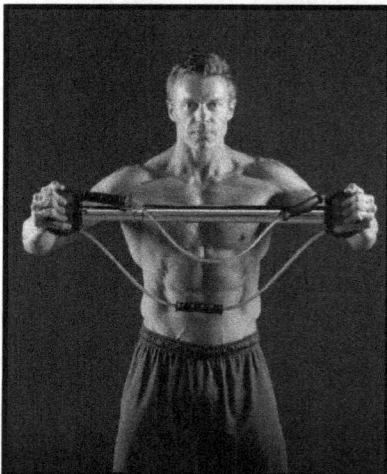

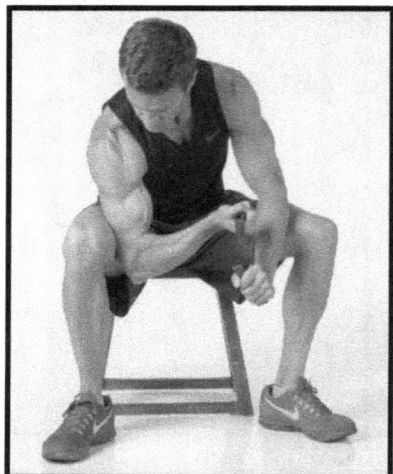

PHASE TEN

07 HYPER-DENSITY X3 METHOD 10,10,7

TUESDAY, THURSDAY, SATURDAY
HOW TO PERFORM THIS ROUTINE: Contract 2 seconds release 2 seconds. Perform 10 reps followed by a 1 second isometric, 10 reps followed by another 1 second isometric, then a final 7 reps. On the 7th rep hold for a 10 second Isometric contraction. Perform 2 rounds. **Perform program for 3 weeks**

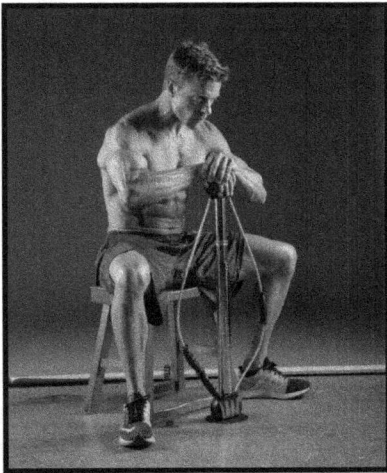

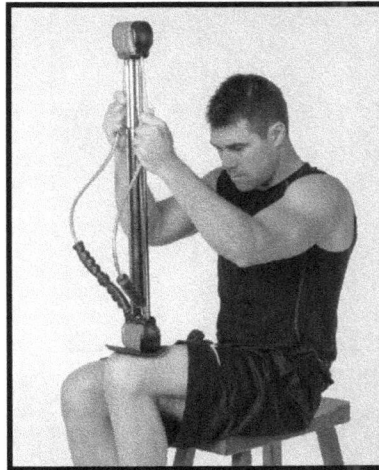

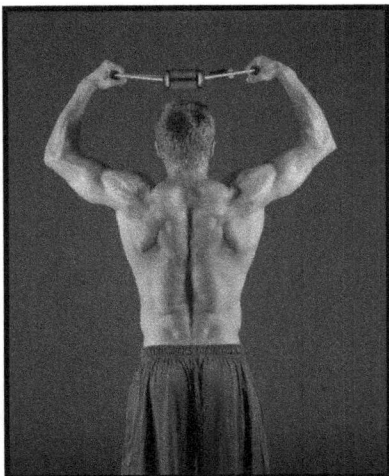

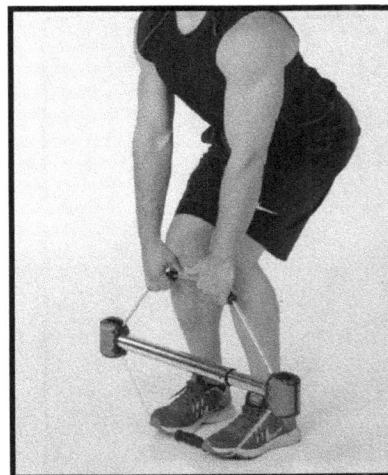

PHASE TEN

07 HYPER-DENSITY X3 METHOD 10,10,7

TUESDAY, THURSDAY, SATURDAY
Routine continued..................

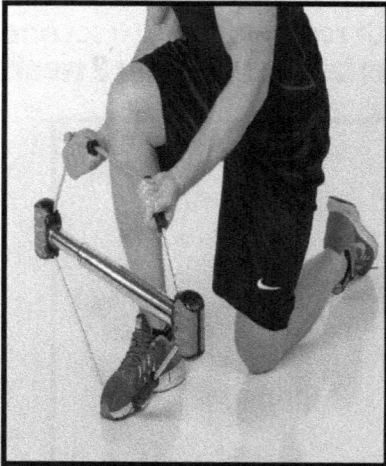

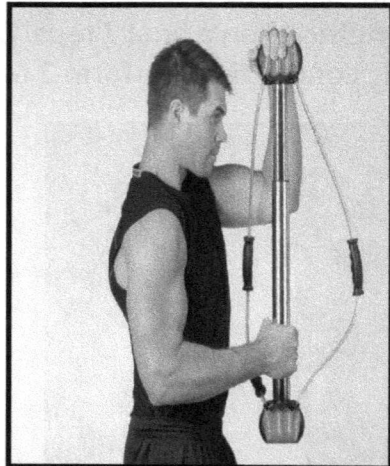

PHASE TEN   TUES, THURS, SAT.

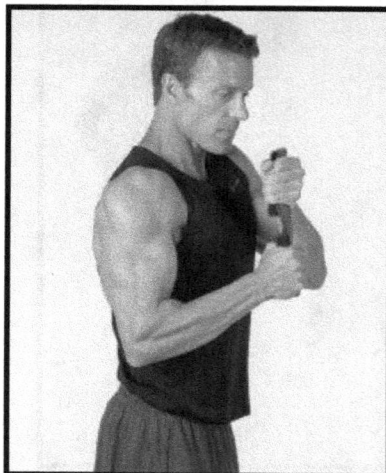

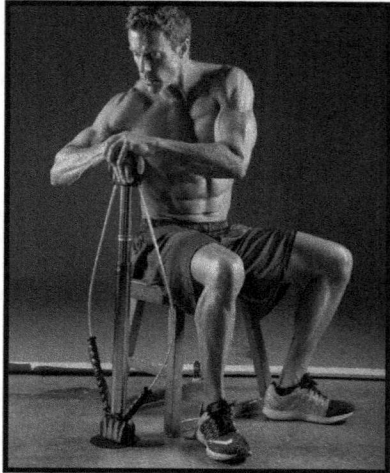

CHAPTER 8
HYPER REP RANGE X1
PHASE 11
3 WEEKS

REP SPEED CONTRACT 2 SECONDS, RELEASE 2 SECONDS

1ST WEEK 20 REPS, 7 SECOND ISOMETRIC...   3 ROUNDS

2ND WEEK 5-7 REPS, 20 SECOND ISOMETRIC.. 3 ROUNDS

3RD WEEK 15 REPS, 10 SECOND ISOMETRIC...   3 ROUNDS

4TH WEEK 30 REPS, 15 SECONDS ISOMETRIC... 3 ROUNDS

HYPER REP RANGE

08 HYPER REP RANGE X1

HOW TO PERFORM THIS ROUTINE:
1ST Week: 20 reps, 7 second Isometric contraction 3 rounds.
2ND Week: 5-7 reps, 20 second Isometric contraction 3 rounds.
3RD Week: 15 reps, 10 second Isometric contraction 3 rounds.
4th Week: 30 reps, 15 second Isometric contraction 3 rounds.

DAY ONE

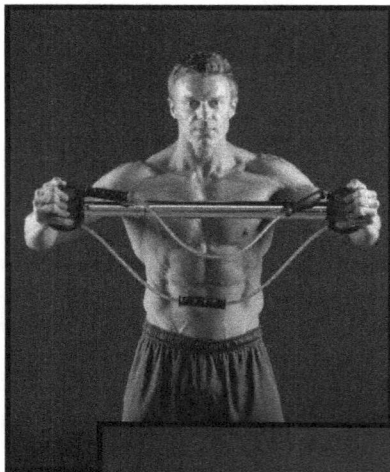
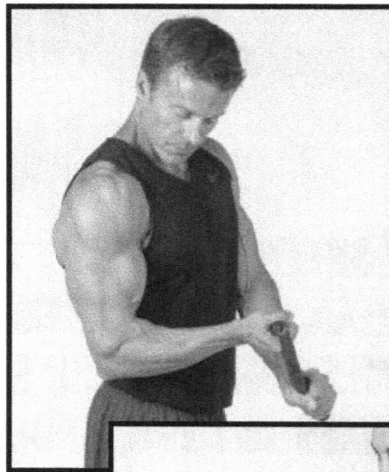
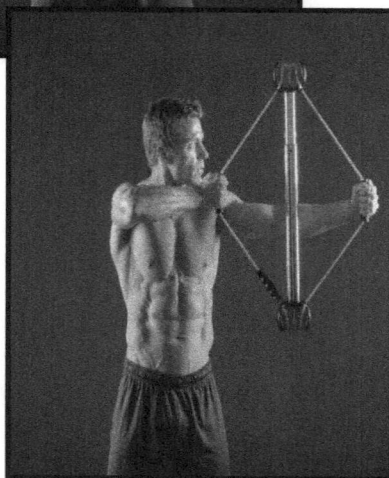
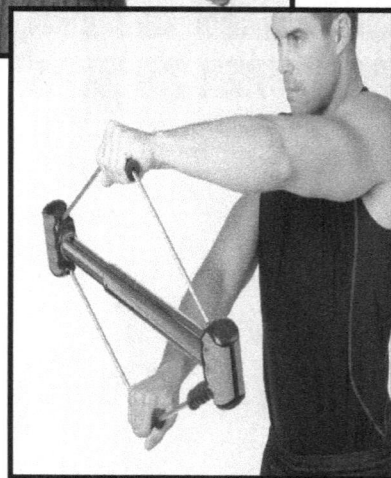

HYPER REP RANGE

08 HYPER REP RANGE X1

HOW TO PERFORM THIS ROUTINE:
1ST Week: 20 reps, 7 second Isometric contraction 3 rounds.
2ND Week: 5-7 reps, 20 second Isometric contraction 3 rounds.
3RD Week: 15 reps, 10 second Isometric contraction 3 rounds.
4th Week: 30 reps, 15 second Isometric contraction 3 rounds.

DAY ONE continued..........

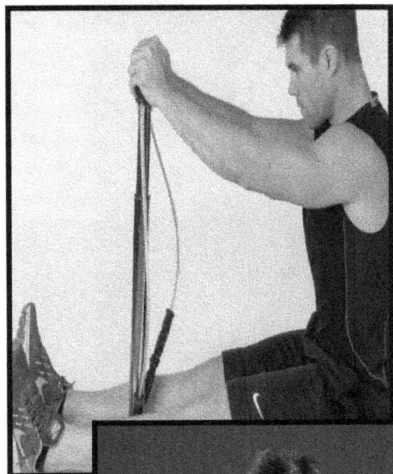

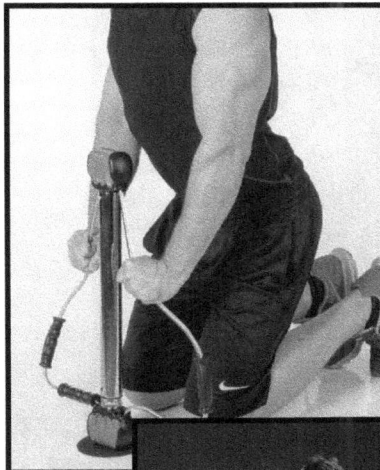

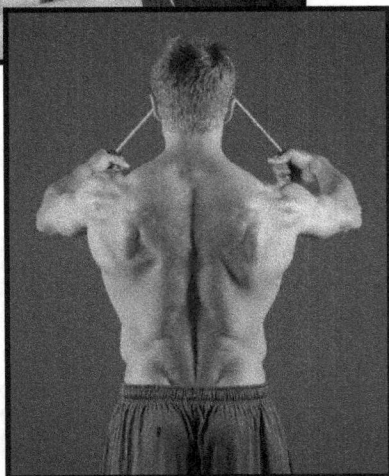

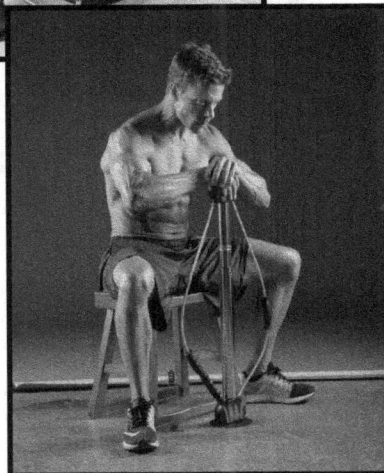

HYPER REP RANGE

08 HYPER REP RANGE X1

HOW TO PERFORM THIS ROUTINE:
1ST Week: 20 reps, 7 second Isometric contraction 3 rounds.
2ND Week: 5-7 reps, 20 second Isometric contraction 3 rounds.
3RD Week: 15 reps, 10 second Isometric contraction 3 rounds.
4th Week: 30 reps, 15 second Isometric contraction 3 rounds.

DAY TWO

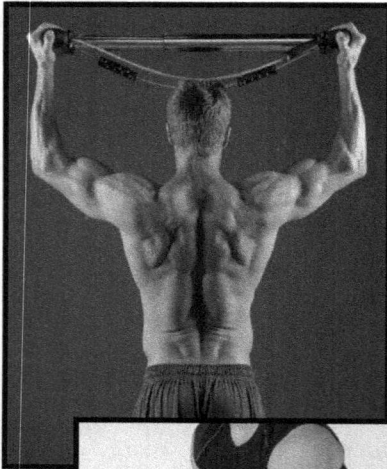
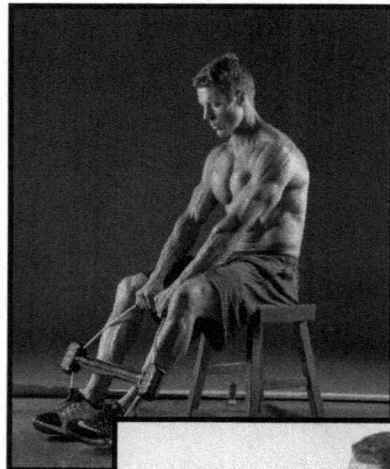
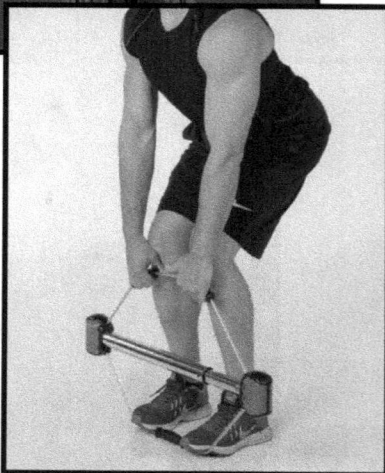
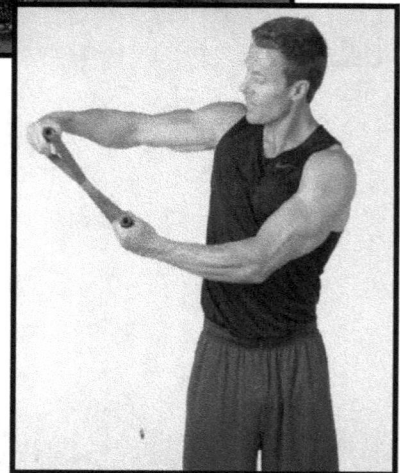

HYPER REP RANGE

08 HYPER REP RANGE X1

HOW TO PERFORM THIS ROUTINE:
1ST Week: 20 reps, 7 second Isometric contraction 3 rounds.
2ND Week: 5-7 reps, 20 second Isometric contraction 3 rounds.
3RD Week: 15 reps, 10 second Isometric contraction 3 rounds.
4th Week: 30 reps, 15 second Isometric contraction 3 rounds.

DAY TWO continued............

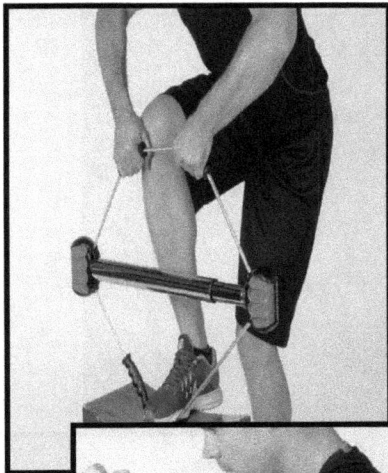

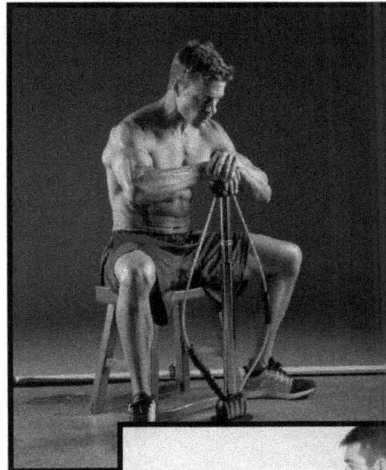

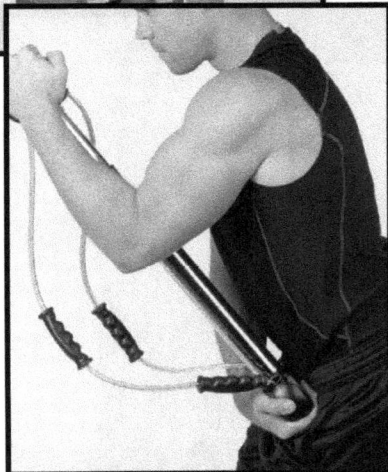

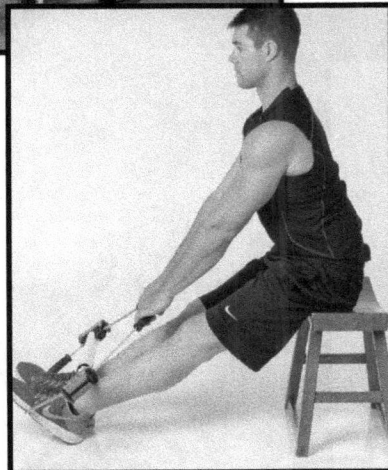

HYPER REP RANGE

08 HYPER REP RANGE X1

HOW TO PERFORM THIS ROUTINE:
1ST Week: 20 reps, 7 second Isometric contraction 3 rounds.
2ND Week: 5-7 reps, 20 second Isometric contraction 3 rounds.
3RD Week: 15 reps, 10 second Isometric contraction 3 rounds.
4th Week: 30 reps, 15 second Isometric contraction 3 rounds.

DAY THREE

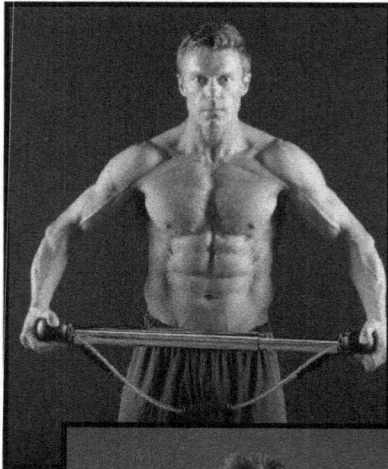
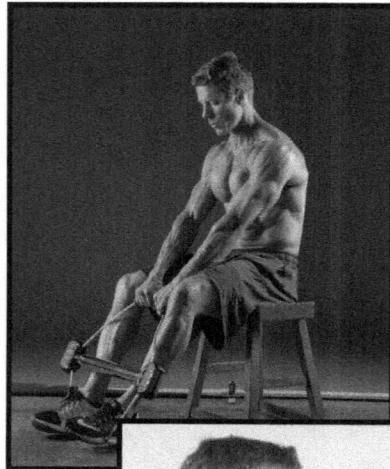
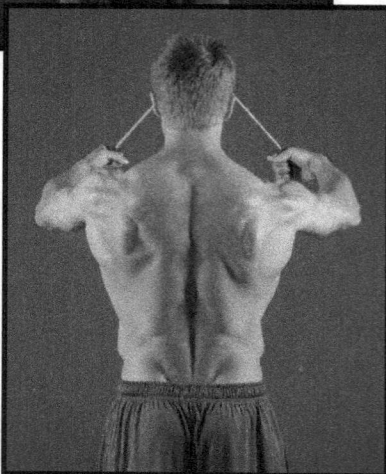
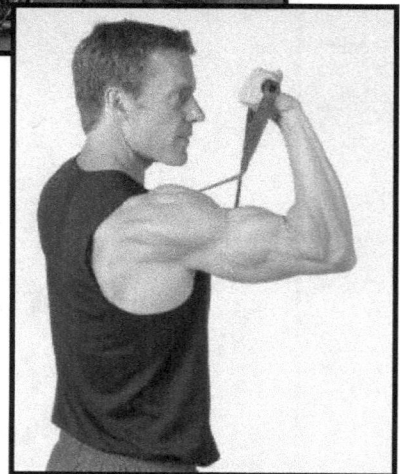

HYPER REP RANGE

08 HYPER REP RANGE X1

HOW TO PERFORM THIS ROUTINE:
1ST Week: 20 reps, 7 second Isometric contraction 3 rounds.
2ND Week: 5-7 reps, 20 second Isometric contraction 3 rounds.
3RD Week: 15 reps, 10 second Isometric contraction 3 rounds.
4th Week: 30 reps, 15 second Isometric contraction 3 rounds.

DAY THREE continued.......

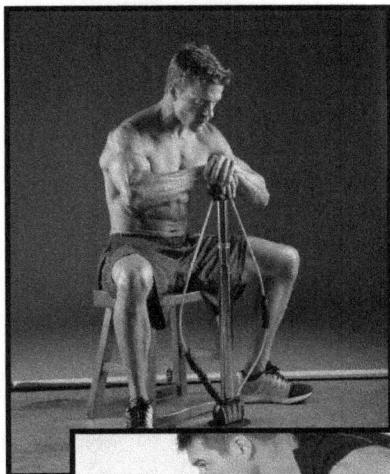
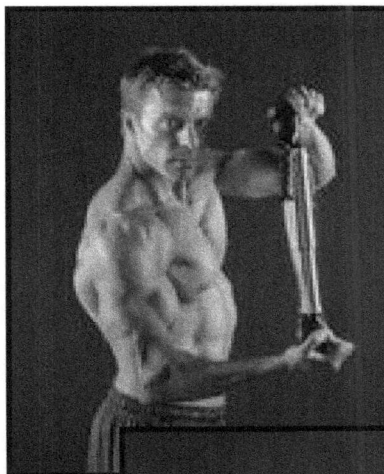
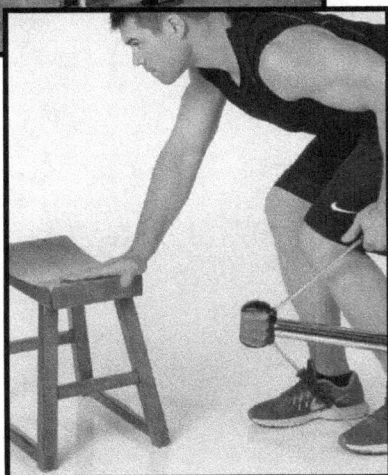
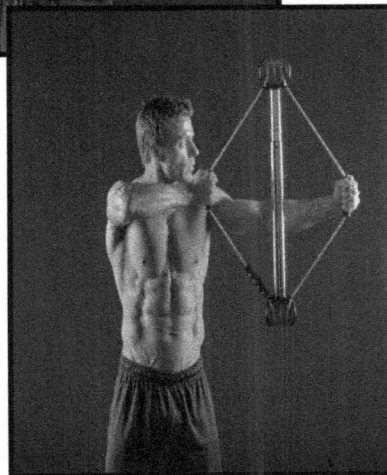

HYPER REP RANGE

08 HYPER REP RANGE X1

HOW TO PERFORM THIS ROUTINE:
1ST Week: 20 reps, 7 second Isometric contraction 3 rounds.
2ND Week: 5-7 reps, 20 second Isometric contraction 3 rounds.
3RD Week: 15 reps, 10 second Isometric contraction 3 rounds.
4th Week: 30 reps, 15 second Isometric contraction 3 rounds.

DAY THREE continued.......

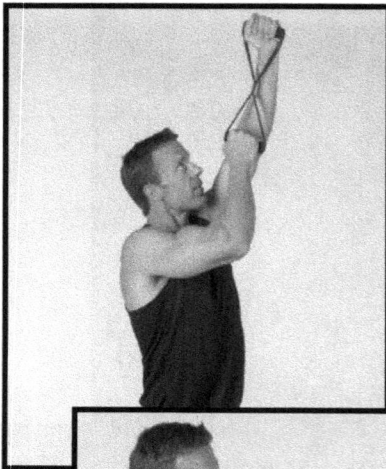

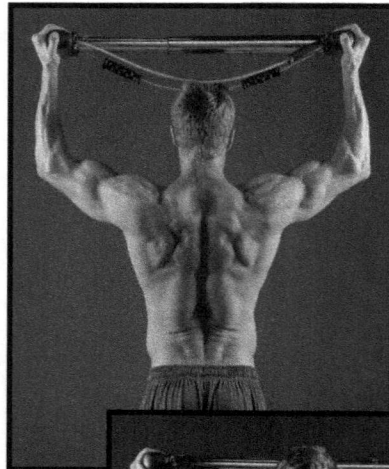

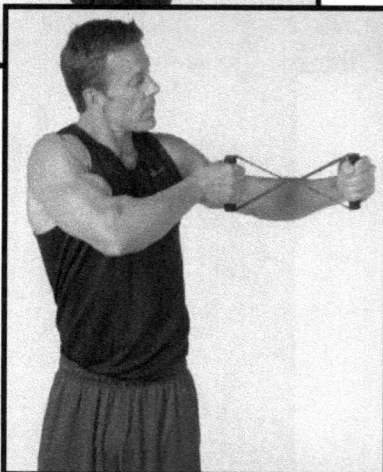

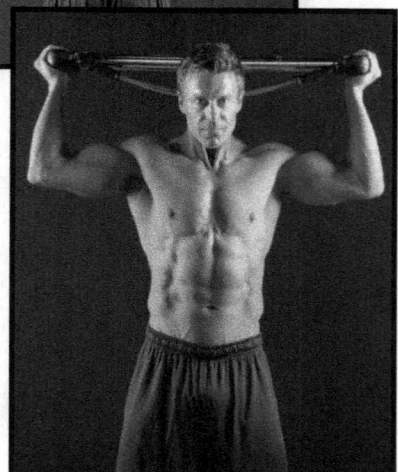

HYPER REP RANGE

08 HYPER REP RANGE X1

HOW TO PERFORM THIS ROUTINE:
1ST Week: 20 reps, 7 second Isometric contraction 3 rounds.
2ND Week: 5-7 reps, 20 second Isometric contraction 3 rounds.
3RD Week: 15 reps, 10 second Isometric contraction 3 rounds.
4th Week: 30 reps, 15 second Isometric contraction 3 rounds.

DAY FOUR

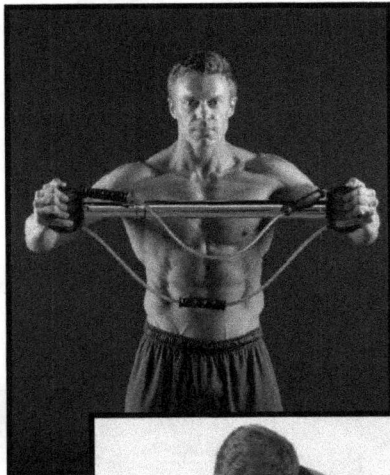
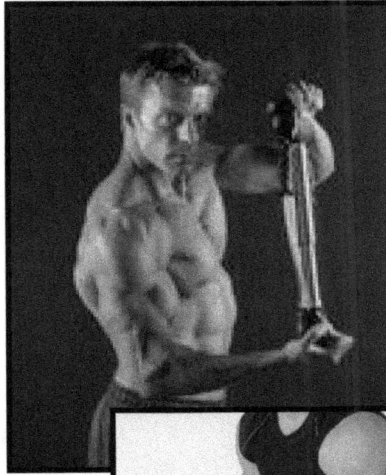
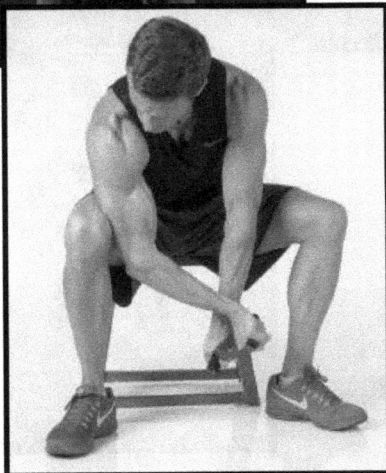
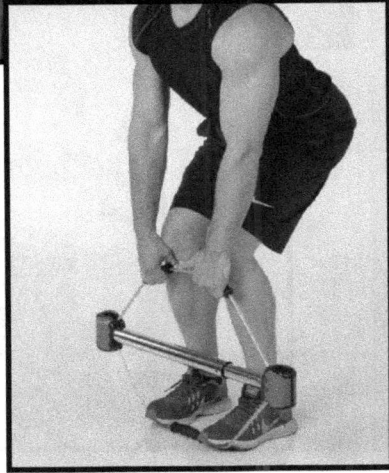

HYPER REP RANGE

08 HYPER REP RANGE X1

HOW TO PERFORM THIS ROUTINE:
1ST Week: 20 reps, 7 second Isometric contraction 3 rounds.
2ND Week: 5-7 reps, 20 second Isometric contraction 3 rounds.
3RD Week: 15 reps, 10 second Isometric contraction 3 rounds.
4th Week: 30 reps, 15 second Isometric contraction 3 rounds.

DAY FOUR continued......

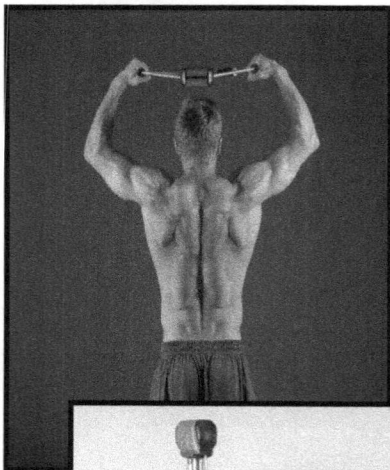

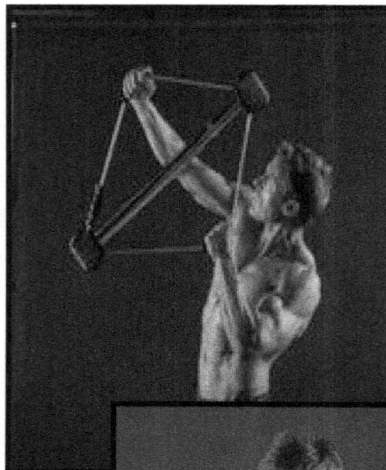

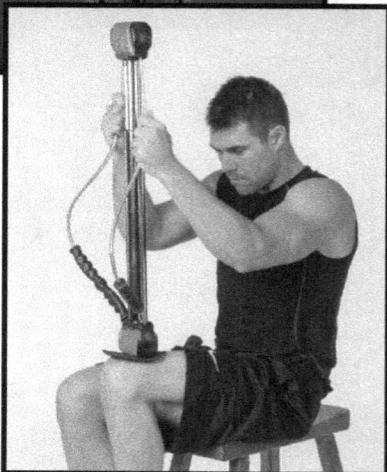

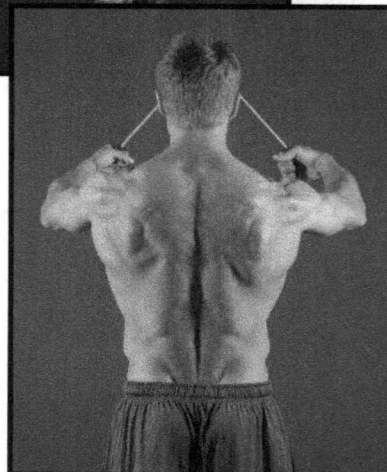

HYPER REP RANGE

08 HYPER REP RANGE X1

HOW TO PERFORM THIS ROUTINE:

1ST Week: 20 reps, 7 second Isometric contraction 3 rounds.
2ND Week: 5-7 reps, 20 second Isometric contraction 3 rounds.
3RD Week: 15 reps, 10 second Isometric contraction 3 rounds.
4th Week: 30 reps, 15 second Isometric contraction 3 rounds.

DAY FIVE

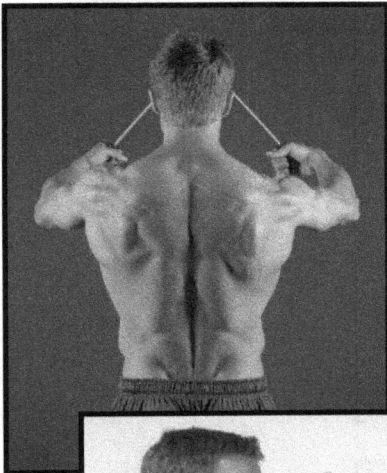
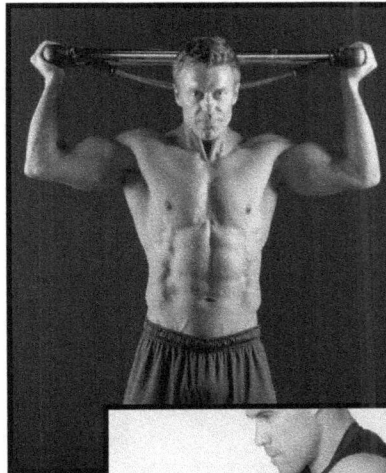
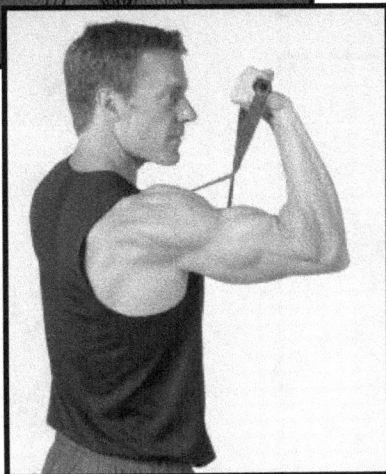
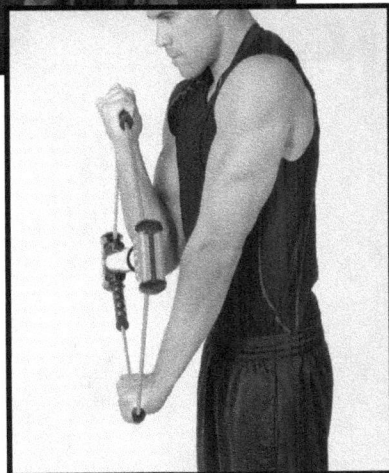

HYPER REP RANGE

08 HYPER REP RANGE X1

HOW TO PERFORM THIS ROUTINE:
1ST Week: 20 reps, 7 second Isometric contraction 3 rounds.
2ND Week: 5-7 reps, 20 second Isometric contraction 3 rounds.
3RD Week: 15 reps, 10 second Isometric contraction 3 rounds.
4th Week: 30 reps, 15 second Isometric contraction 3 rounds.

DAY FIVE continued........

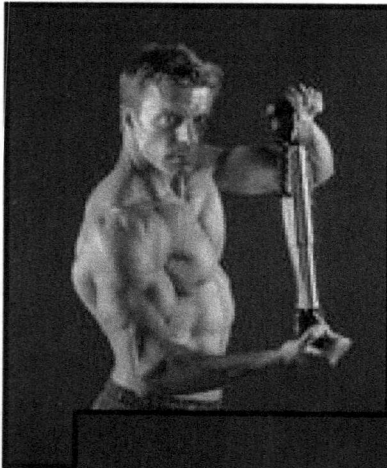

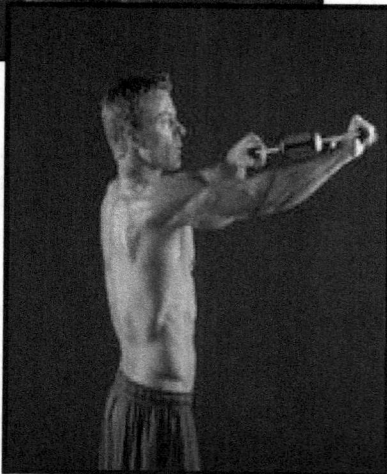

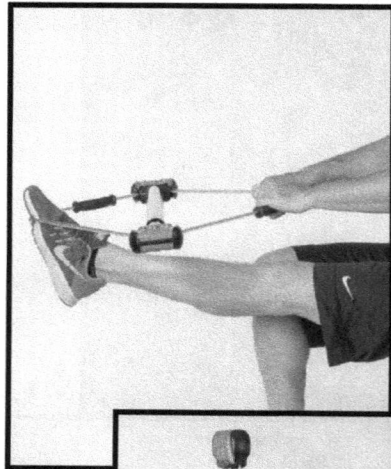

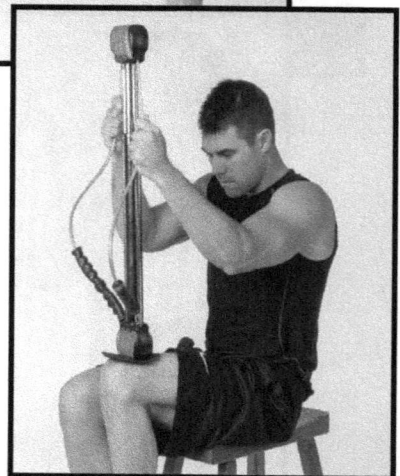

CHAPTER 9
REP RANGE MAX FORCE
MUSCLE-SURGE PROGRAM
PHASE 1
WEEK 1 OF 3
REP SPEED CONTRACT 2 SECONDS, RELEASE 2 SECONDS
PERFORM EACH PHASE TWO WEEKS

MUSCLE-SURGE

09 REP RANGE MAX FORCE

REP RANGE MAX FORCE " MUSCLE-BUILDING PHASE"

WEEK 1: 30x10 Perform 30 reps followed by a 10 second isometric contraction, 2 sets each exercise.

WEEK 2: 10x20 Perform 10 reps followed by a 20 second isometric contraction. 2 sets each exercise.

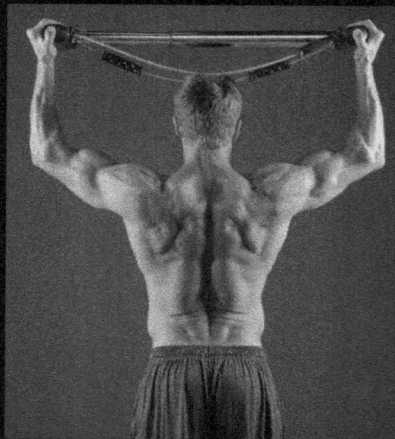

WEEK 3: 20x20 Perform 20 reps followed by a 20 second isometric contraction, 2 sets each exercise.

MUSCLE-SURGE

09 REP RANGE MAX FORCE

HOW TO PERFORM THIS ROUTINE:
WEEK ONE 30x10

Perform 30 reps followed by a 10 second isometric contraction 2 sets each.

DAY ONE

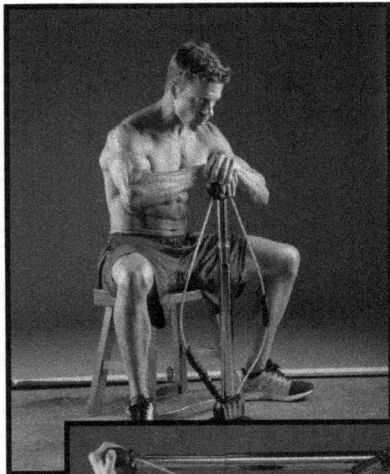
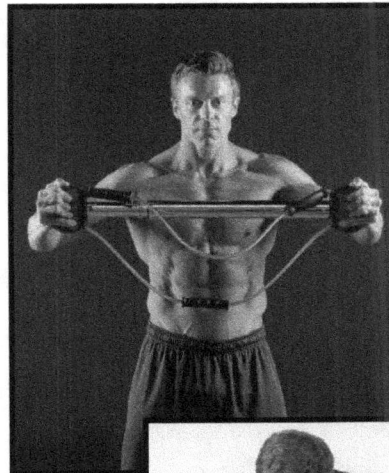
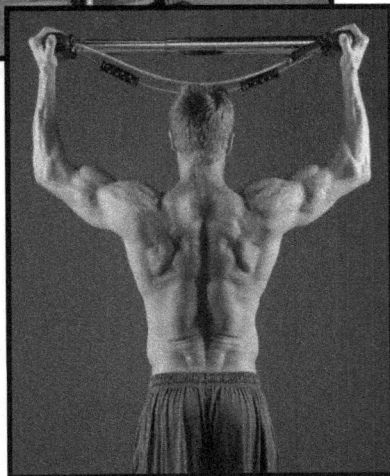
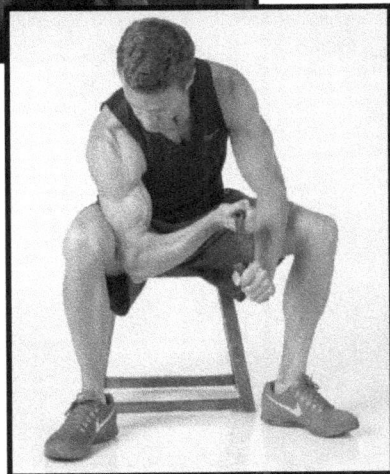

MUSCLE-SURGE

09 REP RANGE MAX FORCE

HOW TO PERFORM THIS ROUTINE:
WEEK ONE 30x10

Perform 30 reps followed by a 10 second isometric contraction 2 sets each.

DAY ONE continued............

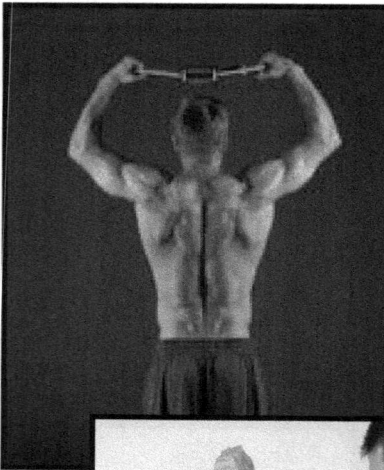

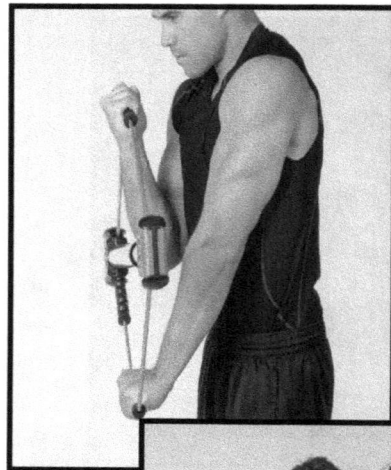

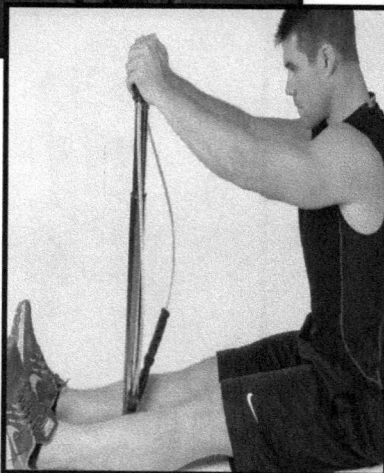

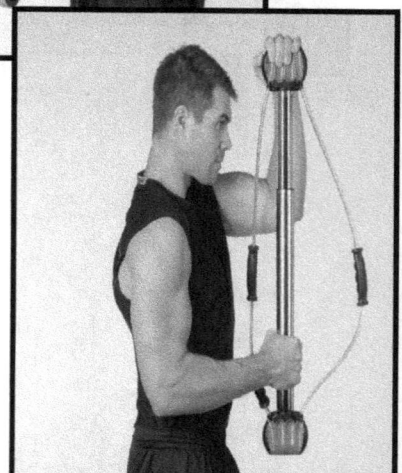

MUSCLE-SURGE

09 REP RANGE MAX FORCE

HOW TO PERFORM THIS ROUTINE:
WEEK ONE 30x10
Perform 30 reps followed by a 10 second isometric contraction 2 sets each.

DAY TWO

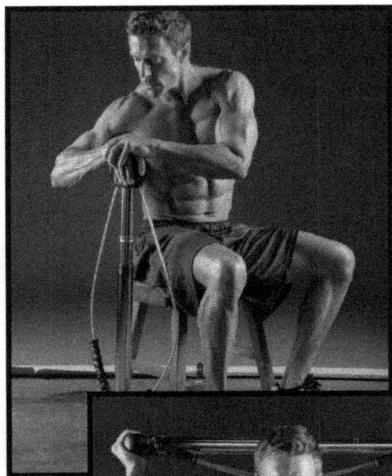
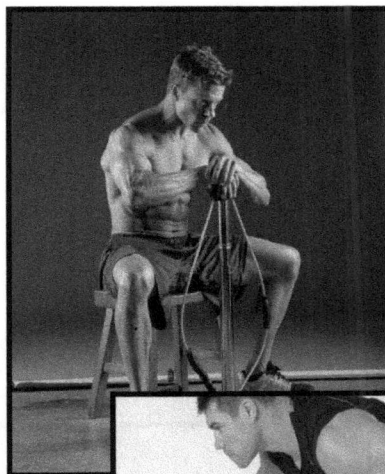
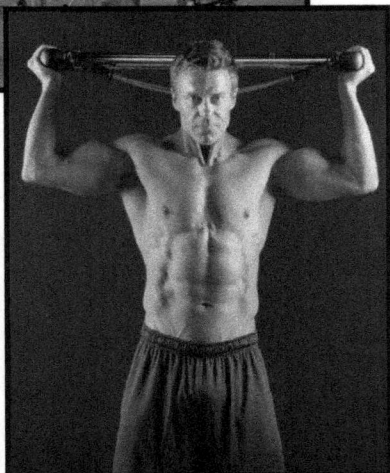
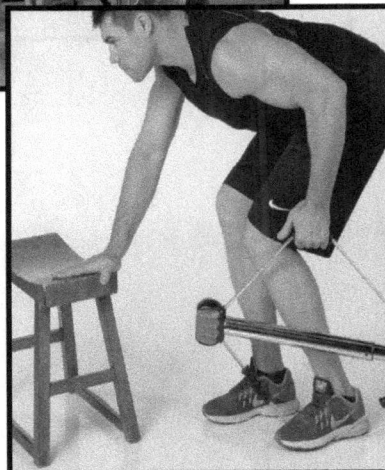

MUSCLE-SURGE

09 REP RANGE MAX FORCE

HOW TO PERFORM THIS ROUTINE:
WEEK ONE 30x10
Perform 30 reps followed by a 10 second isometric contraction 2 sets each.

DAY TWO continued.......

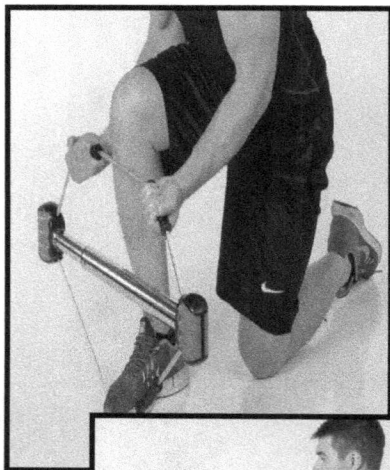

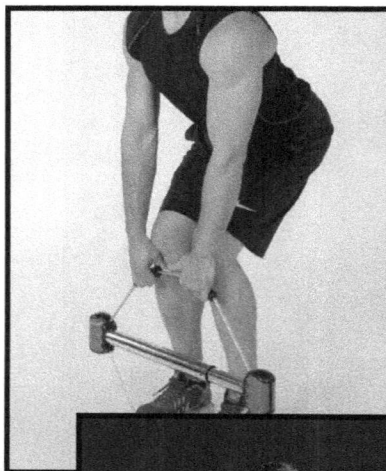

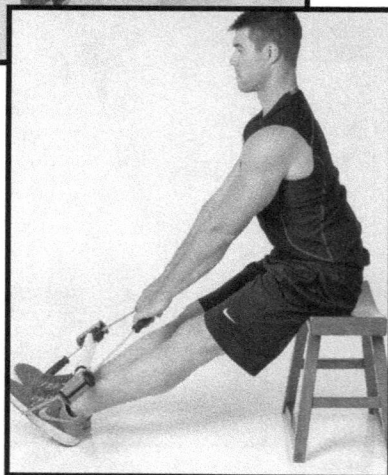

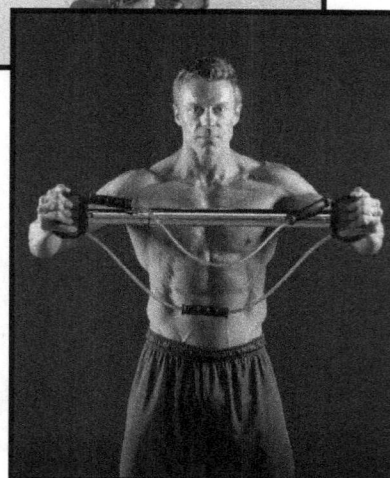

MUSCLE-SURGE

09 REP RANGE MAX FORCE

HOW TO PERFORM THIS ROUTINE:
WEEK ONE 30x10
Perform 30 reps followed by a 10 second isometric contraction 2 sets each.

DAY THREE

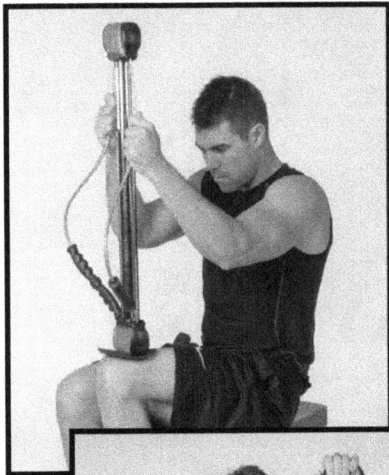
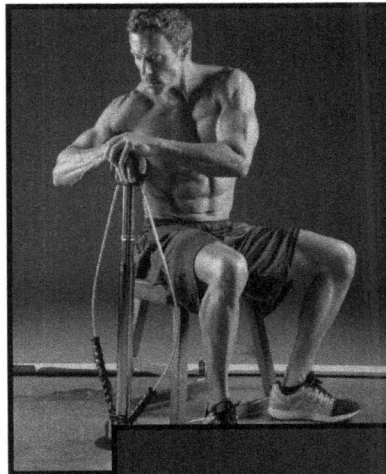
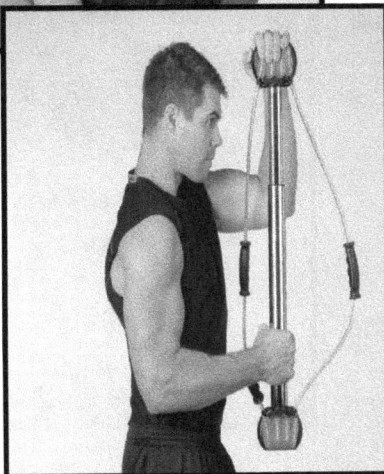
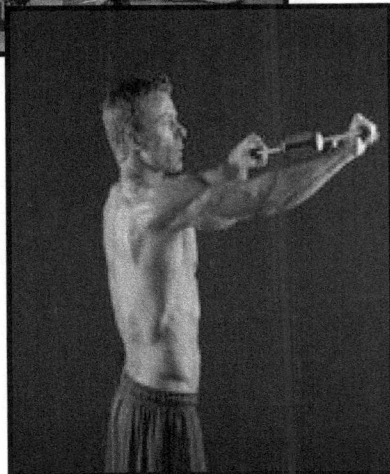

MUSCLE-SURGE

09 REP RANGE MAX FORCE

HOW TO PERFORM THIS ROUTINE:
WEEK ONE 30x10
Perform 30 reps followed by a 10 second isometric contraction 2 sets each.

DAY THREE continued..........

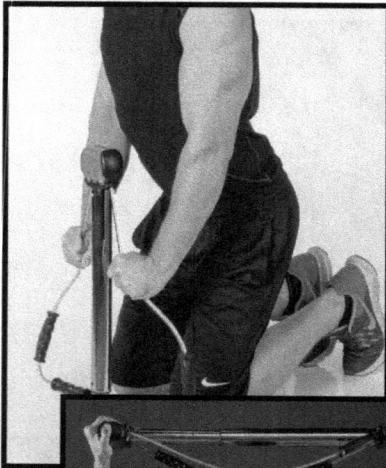

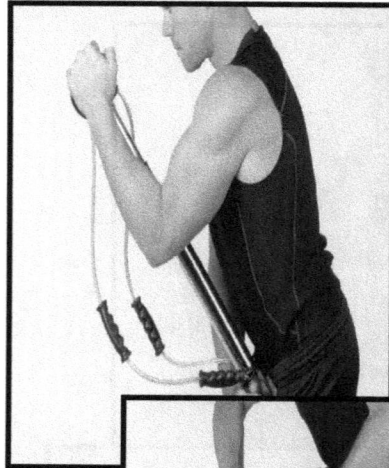

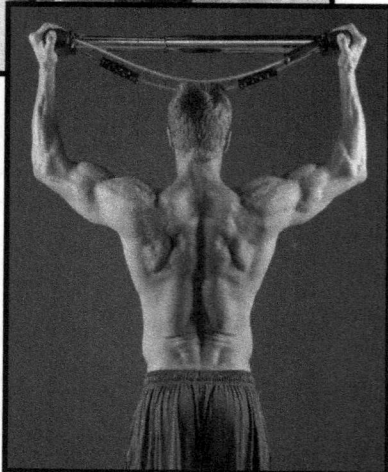

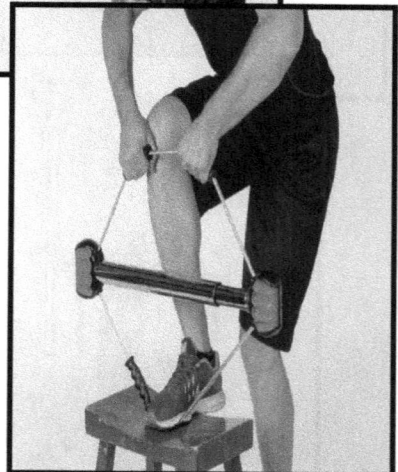

MUSCLE-SURGE

09 REP RANGE MAX FORCE

HOW TO PERFORM THIS ROUTINE:
WEEK ONE 30x10
Perform 30 reps followed by a 10 second isometric contraction 2 sets each.

DAY FOUR

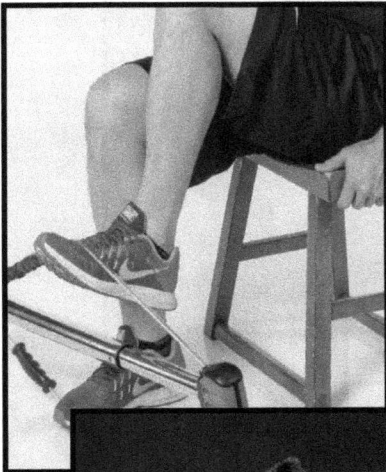

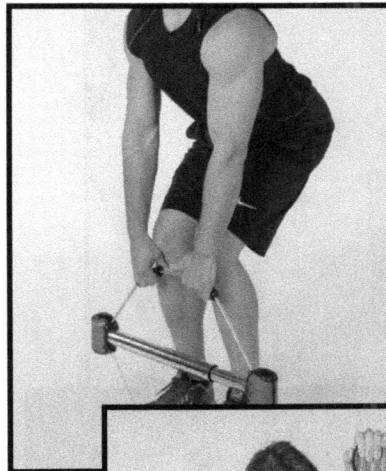

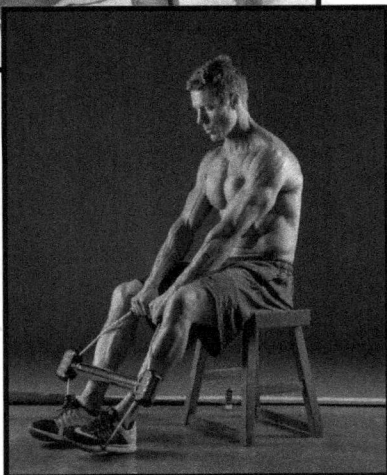

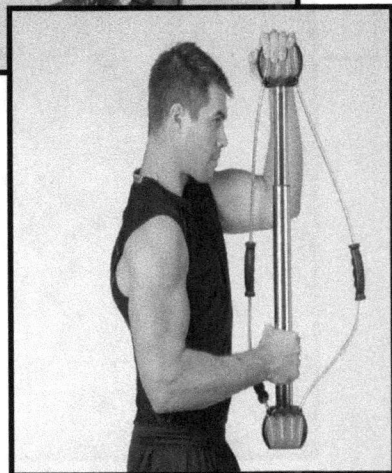

MUSCLE-SURGE

09 REP RANGE MAX FORCE

HOW TO PERFORM THIS ROUTINE:
WEEK ONE 30x10
Perform 30 reps followed by a 10 second isometric contraction 2 sets each.

DAY FOUR continued...........

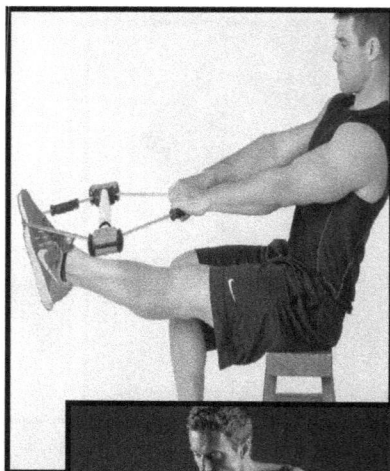

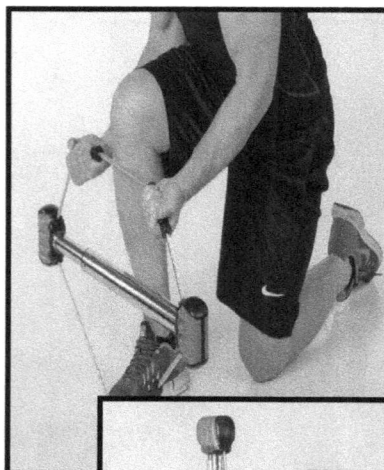

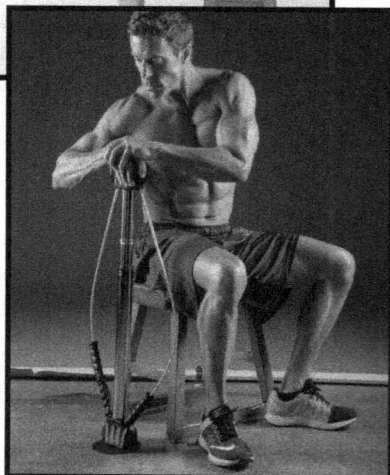

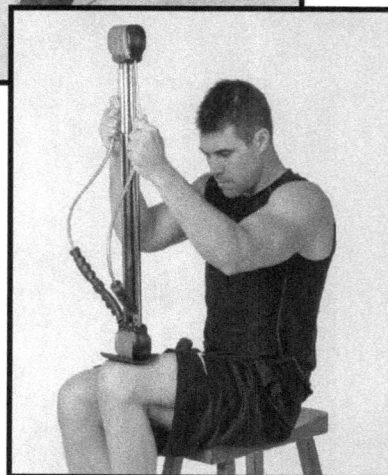

MUSCLE-SURGE

09 REP RANGE MAX FORCE

HOW TO PERFORM THIS ROUTINE:
WEEK ONE 30x10

Perform 30 reps followed by a 10 second isometric contraction 2 sets each.

DAY FIVE

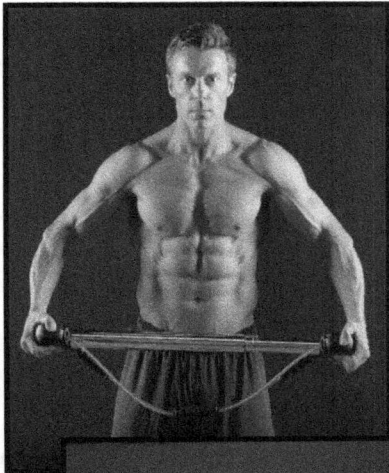

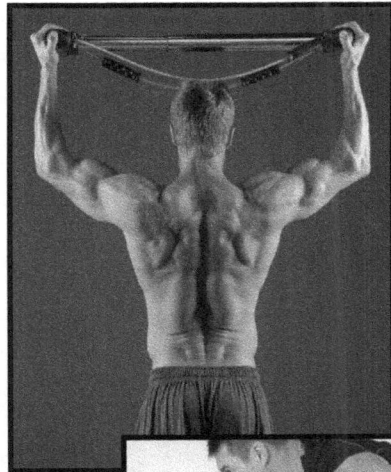

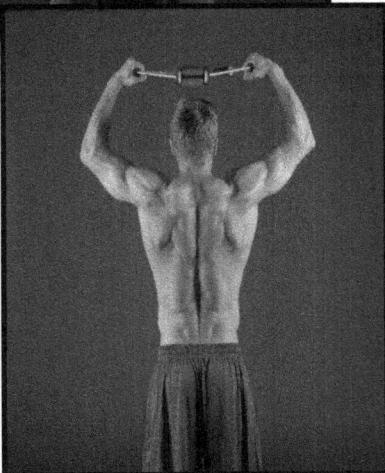

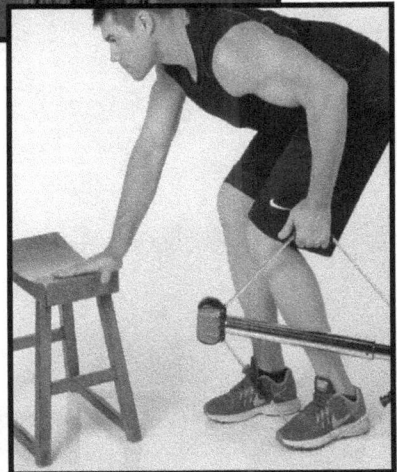

MUSCLE-SURGE

09 REP RANGE MAX FORCE

HOW TO PERFORM THIS ROUTINE:
WEEK ONE 30x10
Perform 30 reps followed by a 10 second isometric contraction 2 sets each.

DAY FIVE continued.............

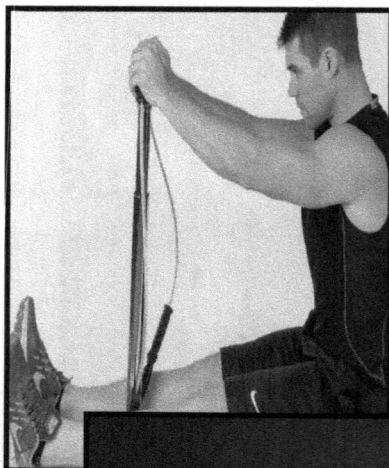

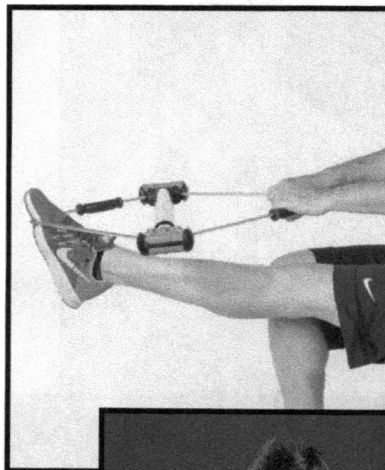

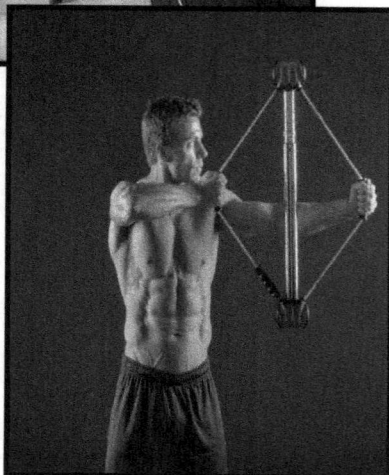

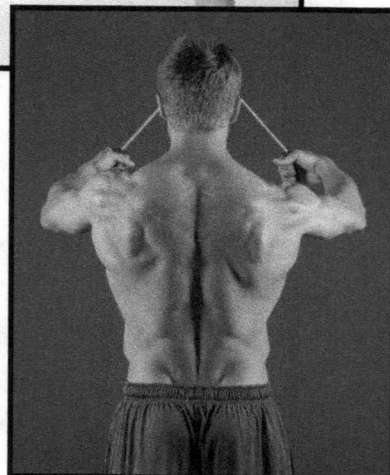

CHAPTER 9

REP RANGE MAX FORCE MUSCLE SURGE

PHASE 2

WEEK 2 OF 3

REP SPEED CONTRACT 2 SECONDS, RELEASE 2 SECONDS

MUSCLE-SURGE

09 REP RANGE MAX FORCE

HOW TO PERFORM THIS ROUTINE:
WEEK TWO 10X20
Perform 10 reps followed by a 20 second isometric contraction, 2 sets.

DAY ONE

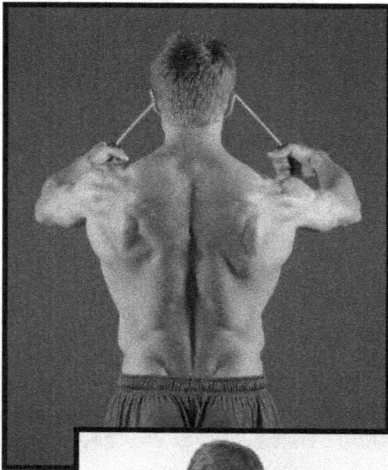
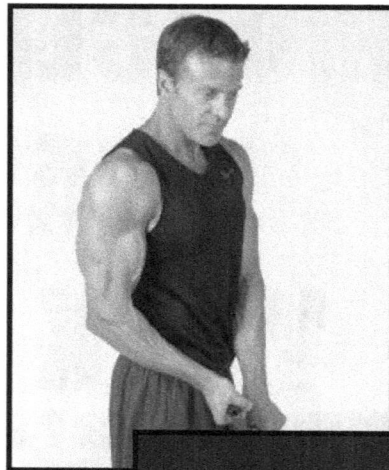
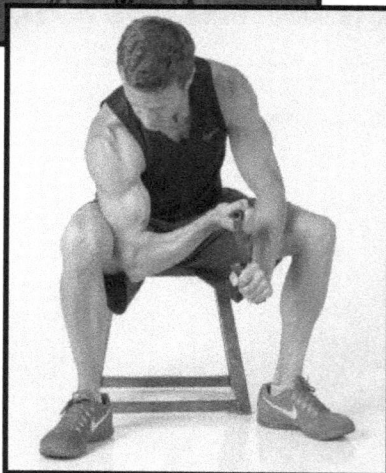
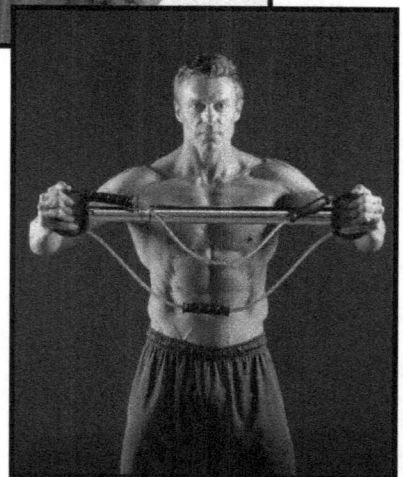

MUSCLE-SURGE

09 REP RANGE MAX FORCE

HOW TO PERFORM THIS ROUTINE:
WEEK TWO 10X20

Perform 10 reps followed by a 20 second isometric contraction, 2 sets.

DAY ONE continued..........

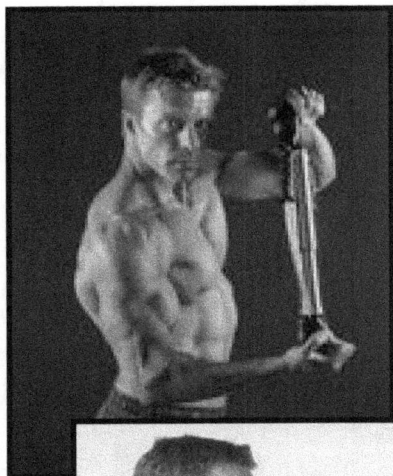
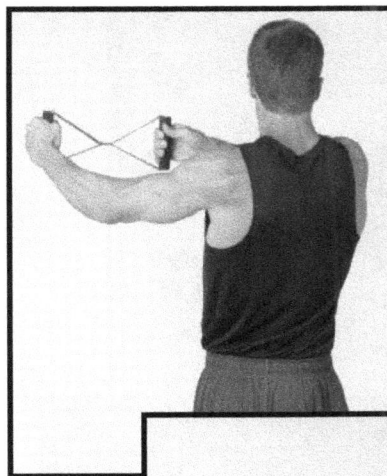
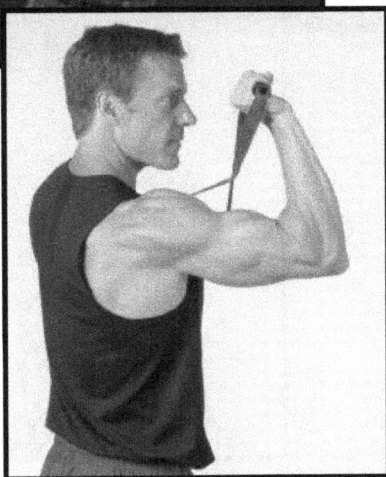
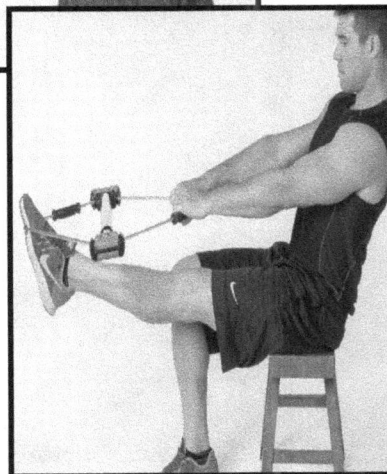

MUSCLE-SURGE

09 REP RANGE MAX FORCE

HOW TO PERFORM THIS ROUTINE:
WEEK TWO 10X20

Perform 10 reps followed by a 20 second isometric contraction, 2 sets.

DAY TWO

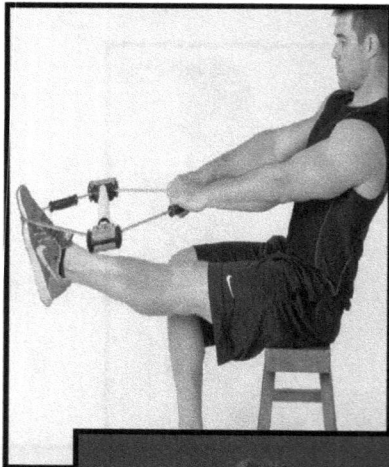

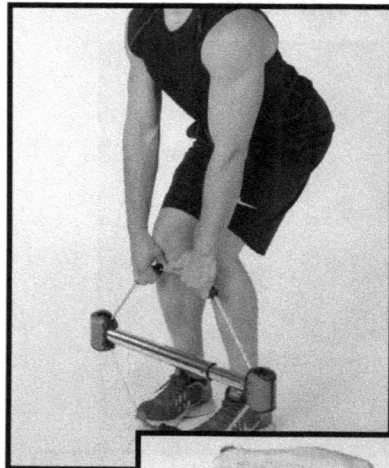

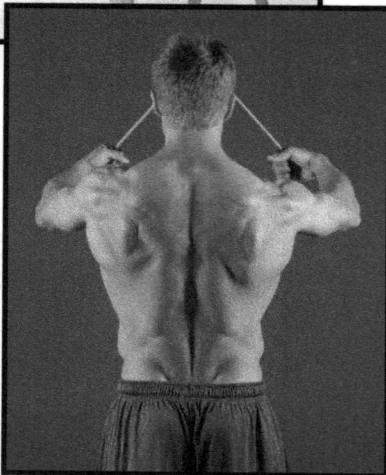

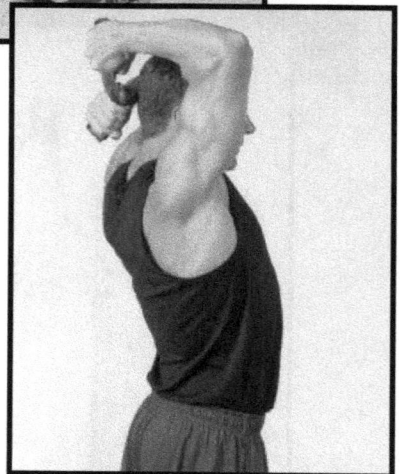

MUSCLE-SURGE

09 REP RANGE MAX FORCE

HOW TO PERFORM THIS ROUTINE:
WEEK TWO 10X20

Perform 10 reps followed by a 20 second isometric contraction, 2 sets.

DAY TWO contin.......

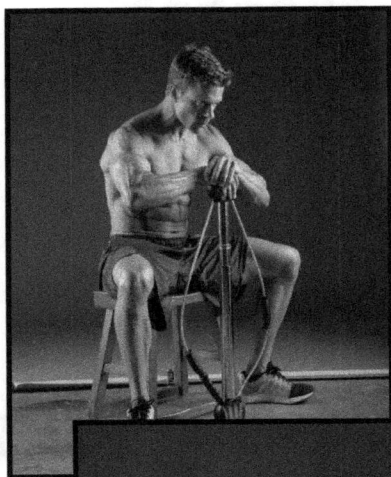

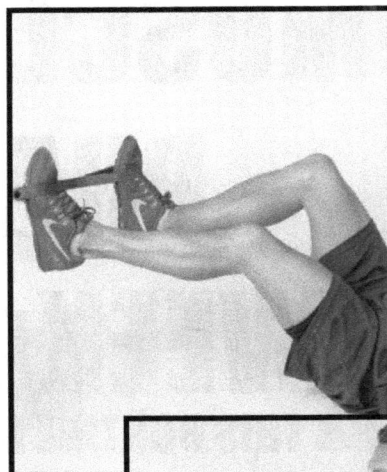

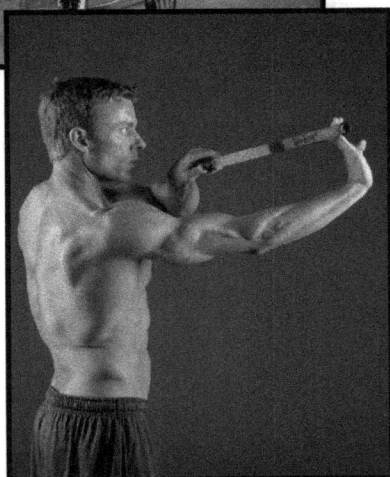

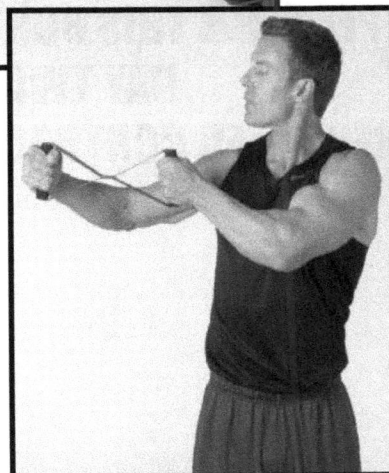

CHAPTER 9
REP RANGE MAX FORCE
MUSCLE-SURGE
PHASE 3
WEEK 3 OF 3

PERFORM THIS ROUTINE BY ALTERNATING DAY ONE AND
DAY TWO FOR 6 DAYS STRAIGHT.
REP SPEED CONTRACT 2 SECONDS, RELEASE 2 SECONDS

MUSCLE-SURGE

09 REP RANGE MAX FORCE

HOW TO PERFORM THIS ROUTINE:
WEEK THREE 20x20

Perform 20 reps followed by a 20 second isometric contraction....2 sets.

DAY ONE

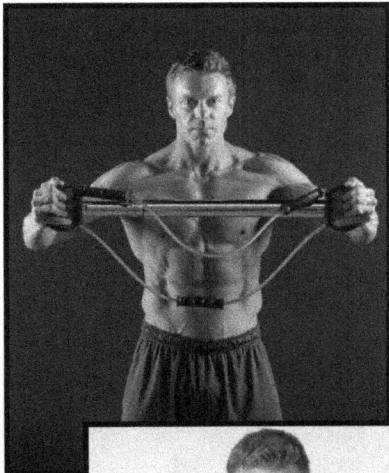

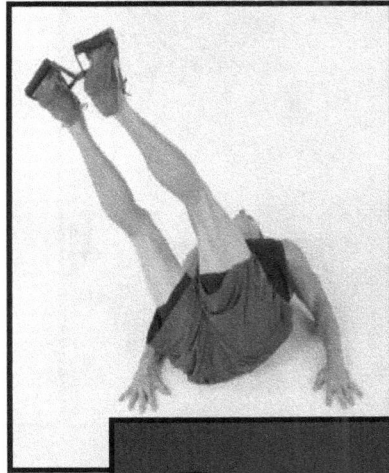

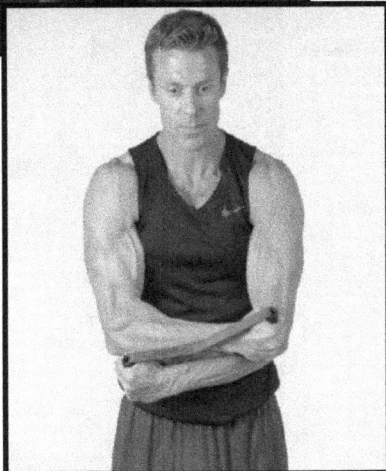

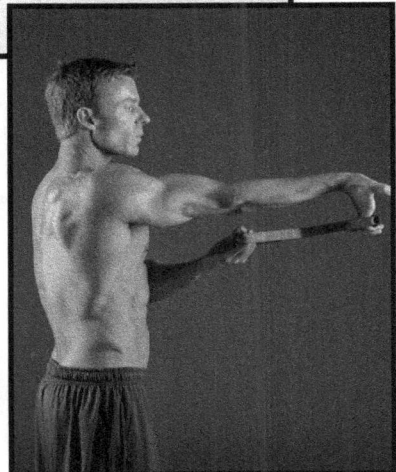

MUSCLE-SURGE

09 REP RANGE MAX FORCE

HOW TO PERFORM THIS ROUTINE:
WEEK THREE 20x20
Perform 20 reps followed by a 20 second isometric contraction....2 sets.

DAY ONE continued............

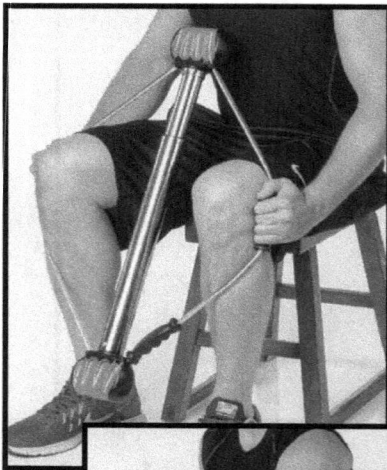

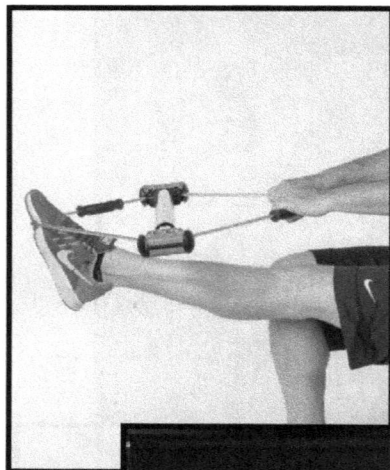

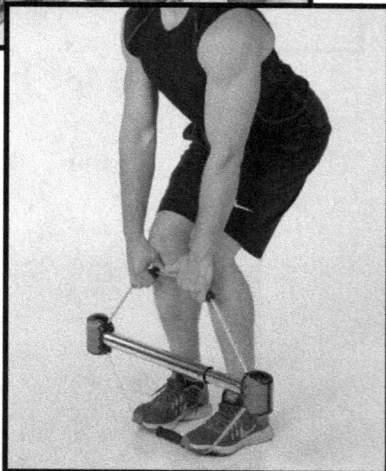

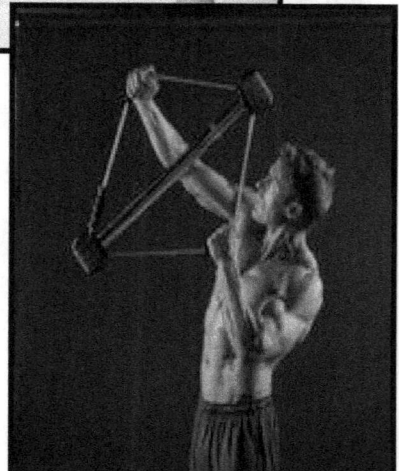

MUSCLE-SURGE

09 REP RANGE MAX FORCE

HOW TO PERFORM THIS ROUTINE:
WEEK THREE 20x20

Perform 20 reps followed by a 20 second isometric contraction....2 sets.

DAY TWO

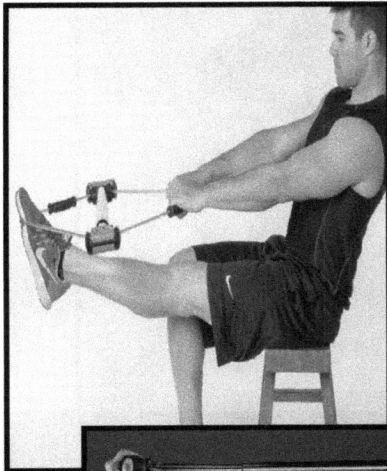

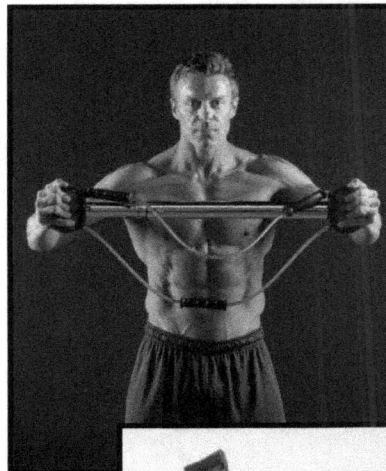

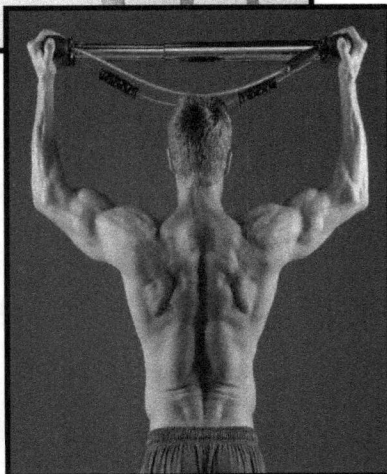

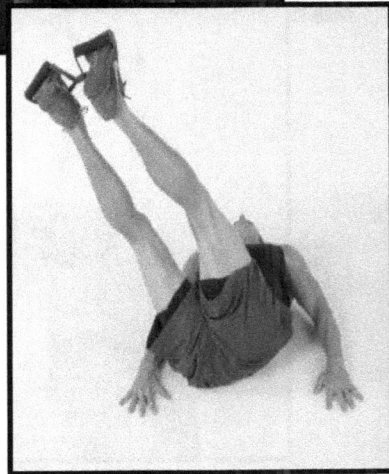

MUSCLE-SURGE

09 REP RANGE MAX FORCE

HOW TO PERFORM THIS ROUTINE:
WEEK THREE 20x20

Perform 20 reps followed by a 20 second isometric contraction....2 sets.

DAY TWO continued..........

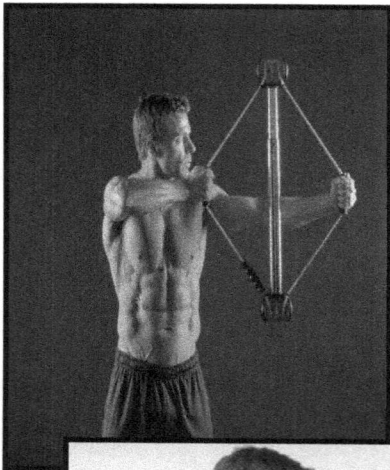

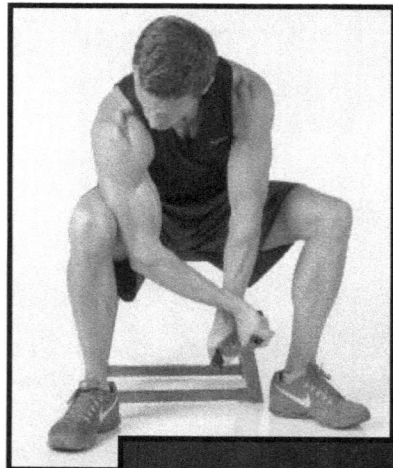

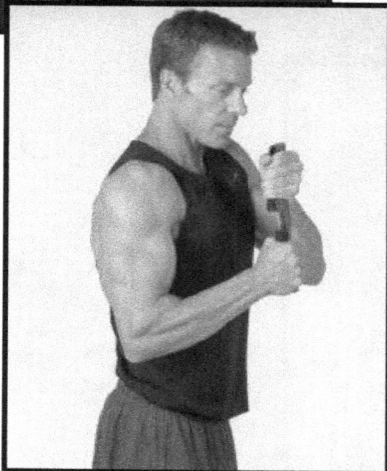

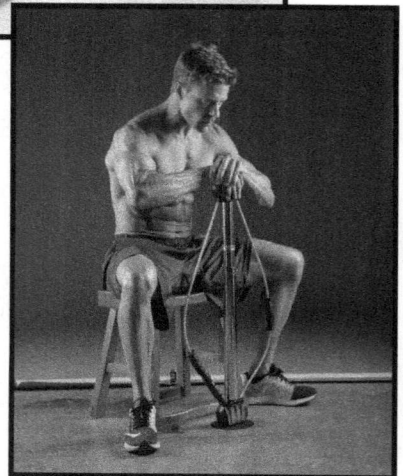

CHAPTER 10

MUSCLE-SURGE
ENDURANCE FX9
PHASE 13

PERFORM THIS PHASE FOR 4 WEEKS

MUSCLE-SURGE

10 ENDURANCE FX9

HOW TO PERFORM THIS ROUTINE:
ENDURANCE FX9

Perform the **ENDURANCE FX9 WORKOUT**—by performing 30 reps. Perform all exercises one after the other until all exercises are completed without rest. Perform 2 rounds of these between each round rest for 5 seconds before starting another round.
Alternate day one and day two for 6 days per week.

DAY ONE

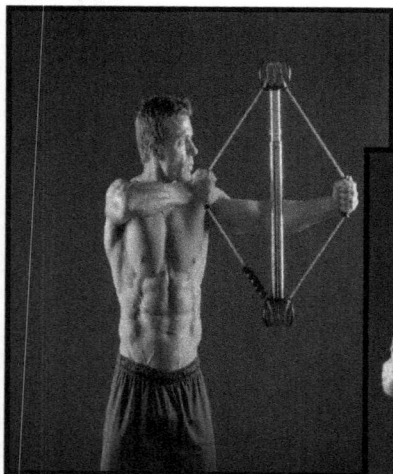
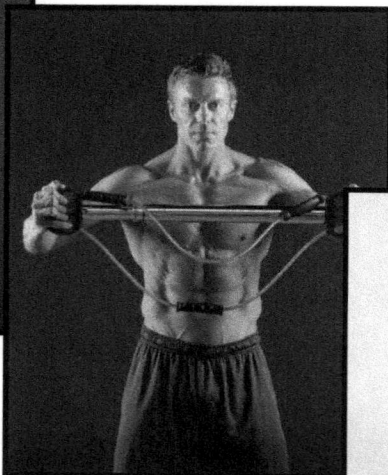
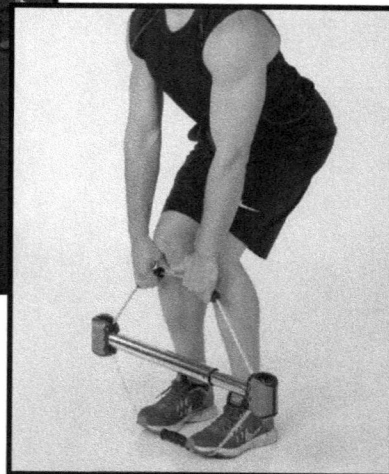

MUSCLE-SURGE

10 ENDURANCE FX9

HOW TO PERFORM THIS ROUTINE:
ENDURANCE FX9

Perform the **ENDURANCE FX9 WORKOUT**—by performing 30 reps. Perform all exercises one after the other until all exercises are completed without rest. Perform 2 rounds of these between each round rest for 5 seconds before starting another round.
Alternate day one and day two for 6 days per week.

DAY ONE continued.........

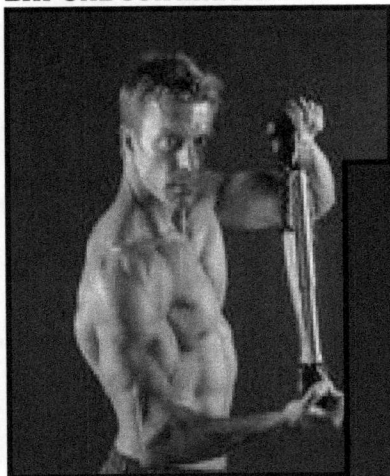

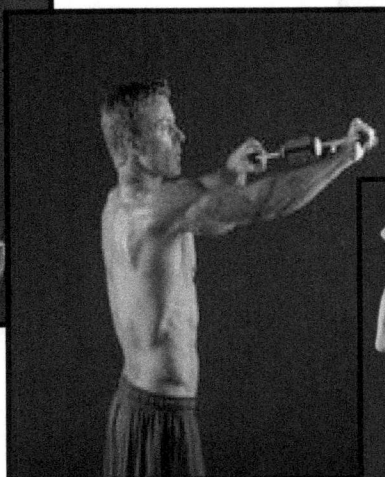

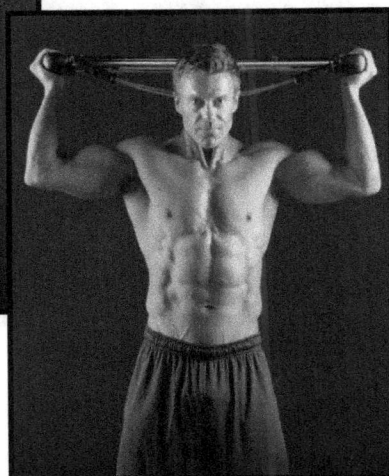

MUSCLE-SURGE

10 ENDURANCE FX9

HOW TO PERFORM THIS ROUTINE:
ENDURANCE FX9

Perform the **ENDURANCE FX9 WORKOUT**—by performing 30 reps. Perform all exercises one after the other until all exercises are completed without rest. Perform 2 rounds of these between each round rest for 5 seconds before starting another round.
Alternate day one and day two for 6 days per week.

DAY ONE continued......

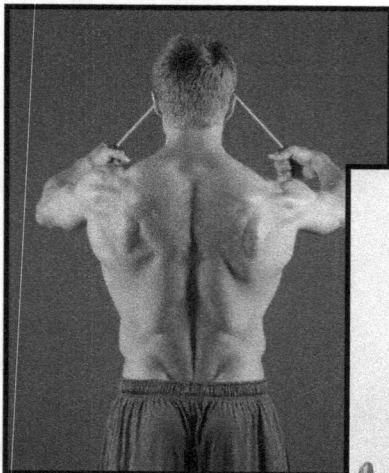

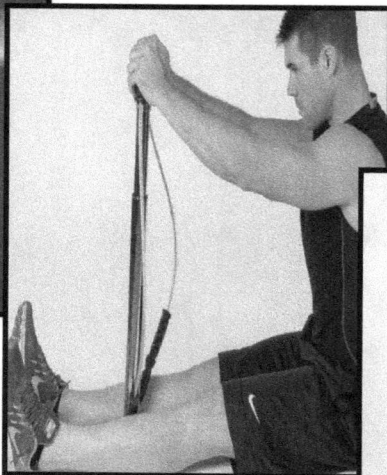

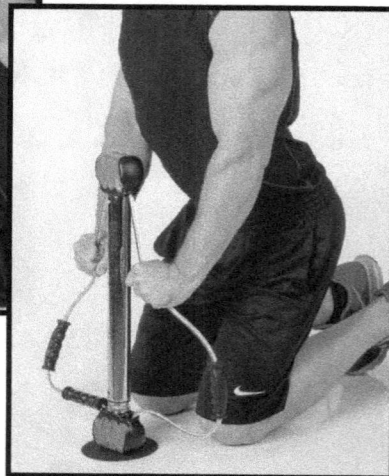

MUSCLE-SURGE

10 ENDURANCE FX9

HOW TO PERFORM THIS ROUTINE:
ENDURANCE FX9

Perform the **ENDURANCE FX9 WORKOUT**—by performing 30 reps. Perform all exercises one after the other until all exercises are completed without rest. Perform 2 rounds of these between each round rest for 5 seconds before starting another round.
Alternate day one and day two for 6 days per week.

DAY TWO

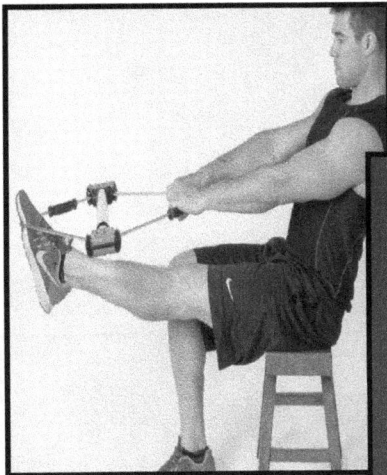
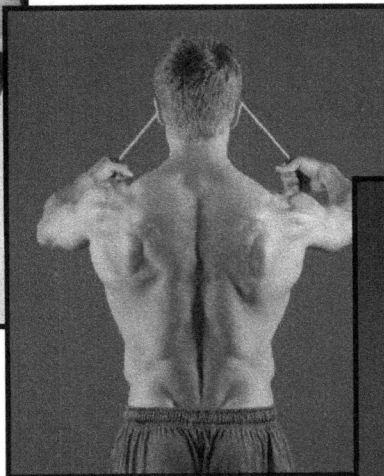
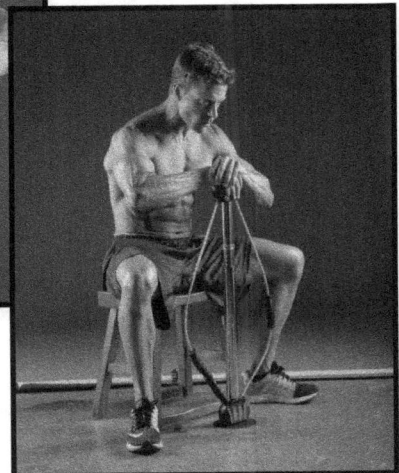

MUSCLE-SURGE

10 ENDURANCE FX9

HOW TO PERFORM THIS ROUTINE:
ENDURANCE FX9

Perform the **ENDURANCE FX9 WORKOUT**—by performing 30 reps. Perform all exercises one after the other until all exercises are completed without rest. Perform 2 rounds of these between each round rest for 5 seconds before starting another round.
Alternate day one and day two for 6 days per week.

DAY TWO continue........

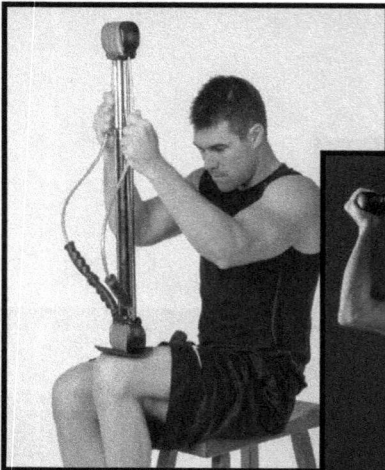

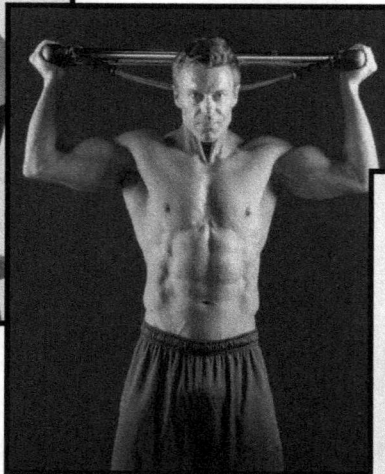

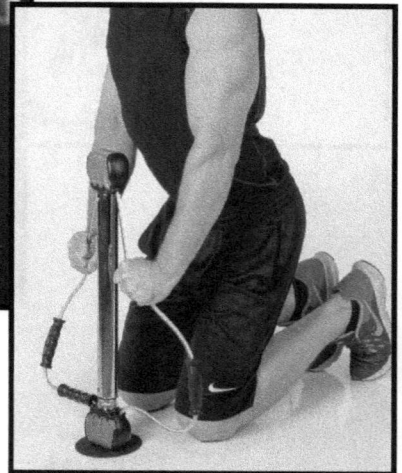

MUSCLE-SURGE

10 POWER 7 PROGRAM

HOW TO PERFORM THIS ROUTINE:
ENDURANCE FX9

Perform the **ENDURANCE FX9 WORKOUT**—by performing 30 reps. Perform all exercises one after the other until all exercises are completed without rest. Perform 2 rounds of these between each round rest for 5 seconds before starting another round.
Alternate day one and day two for 6 days per week.

DAY TWO continued..........

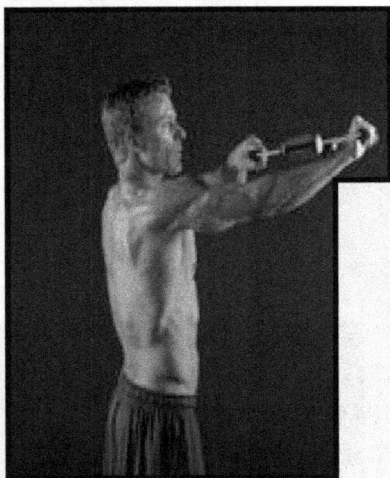

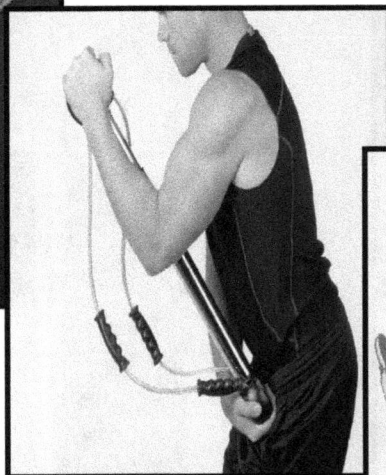

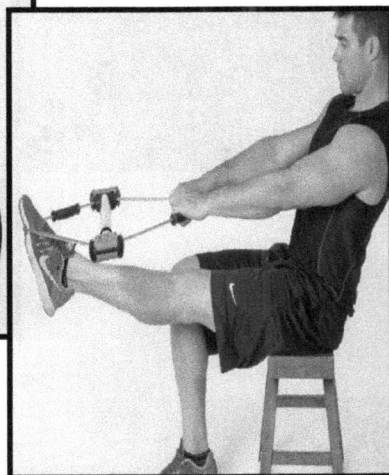

MUSCLE-SURGE

10 ENDURANCE FX9

HOW TO PERFORM THIS ROUTINE:
ENDURANCE FX9

Perform the **ENDURANCE FX9 WORKOUT**—by performing 30 reps. Perform all exercises one after the other until all exercises are completed without rest. Perform 2 rounds of these between each round rest for 5 seconds before starting another round.
Alternate day one and day two for 6 days per week.

DAY TWO continued...........

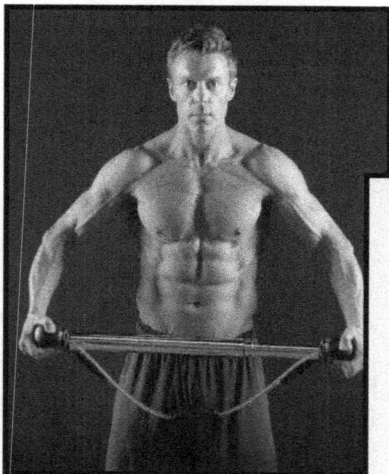

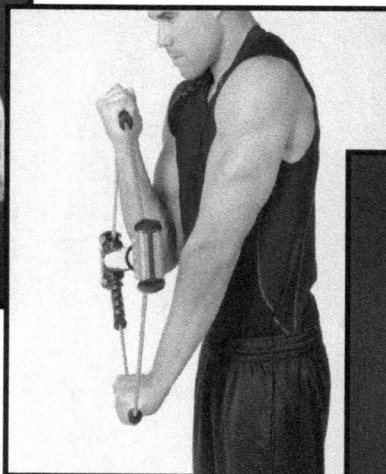

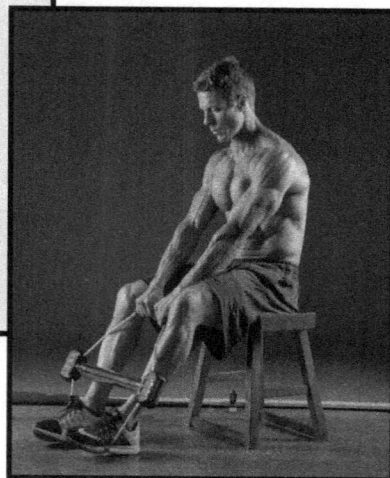

CHAPTER 11
REP RANGE MAX X4
MUSCLE-SURGE
PHASE ONE

REP RANGES CHANGE THROUGHOUT THE WEEK

REP RANGE MAX X4

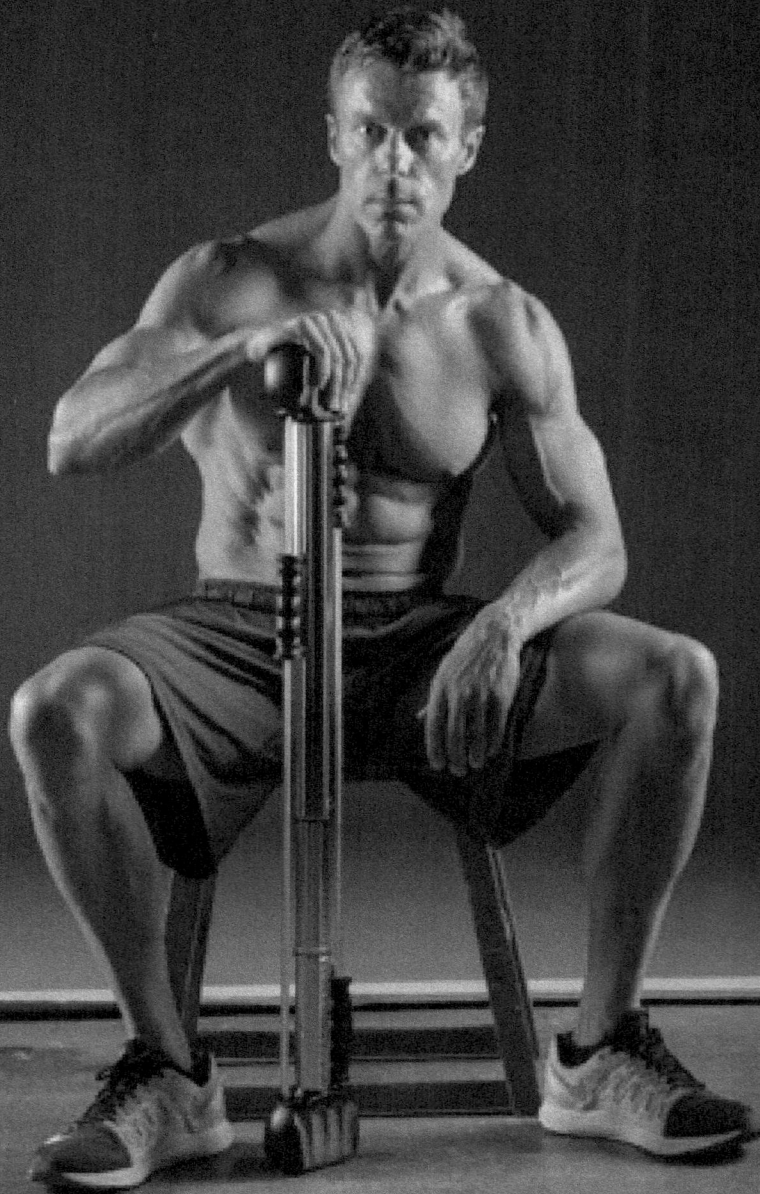

REP RANGE MAX X4

11 REP RANGE MAX X4 PHASE ONE

HOW TO PERFORM THIS ROUTINE:
REP RANGE MAX X2

Day 1=5-7 reps, Day 2=10 reps, Day 3=20 reps, Day 4=20 reps, Day 5=30 reps
Day 6=40 reps, Day 7=10 reps. On the last rep perform a 10 second
Isometric contraction. Perform all exercises without rest for 2 rounds.
Perform this routine every day 7 days per week for 2 weeks

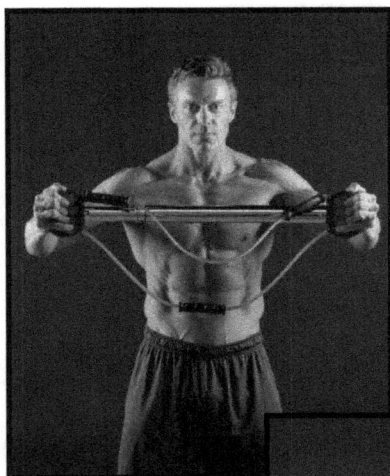

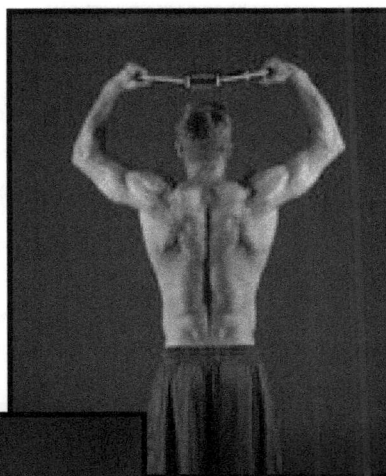

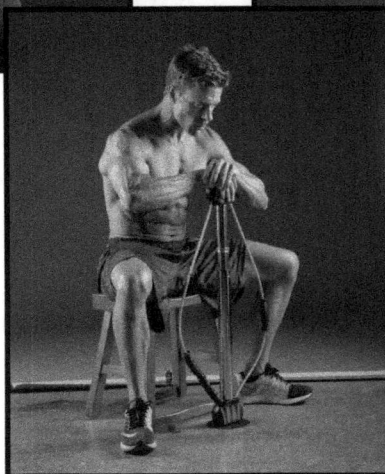

REP RANGE MAX X4

11 REP RANGE MAX X4 PHASE ONE

HOW TO PERFORM THIS ROUTINE:
REP RANGE MAX X2

Day 1=5-7 reps, Day 2=10 reps, Day 3=20 reps, Day 4=20 reps, Day 5=30 reps Day 6=40 reps, Day 7=10 reps. On the last rep perform a 10 second Isometric contraction. Perform all exercises without rest for 2 rounds.
Perform this routine every day 7 days per week for 2 weeks

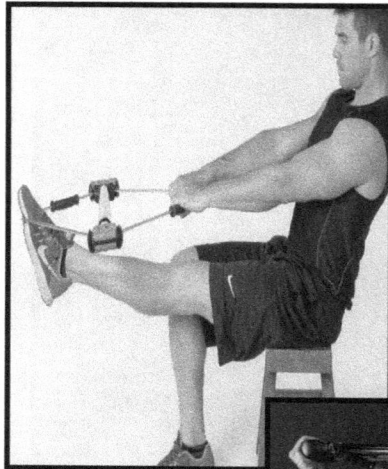

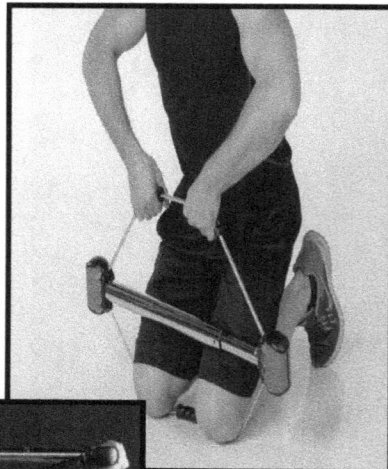

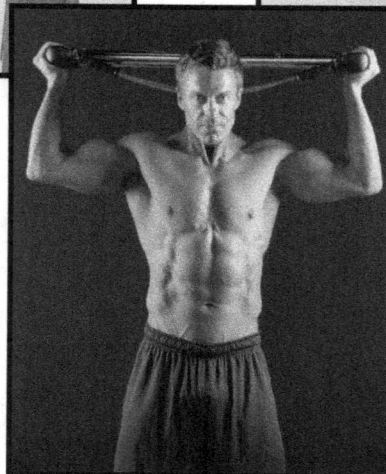

REP RANGE MAX X4

11 REP RANGE MAX X4 PHASE ONE

HOW TO PERFORM THIS ROUTINE:
REP RANGE MAX X2

Day 1=5-7 reps, Day 2=10 reps, Day 3=20 reps, Day 4=20 reps, Day 5=30 reps Day 6=40 reps, Day 7=10 reps. On the last rep perform a 10 second Isometric contraction. Perform all exercises without rest for 2 rounds.
Perform this routine every day 7 days per week for 2 weeks

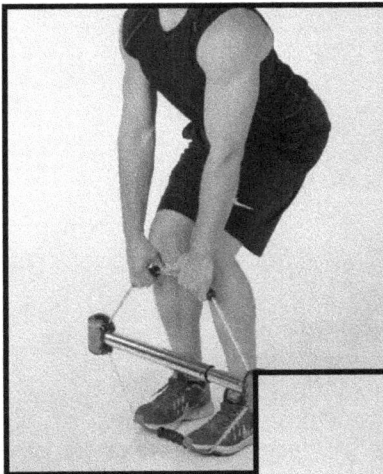
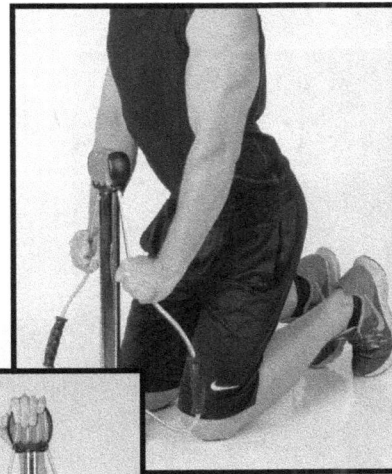
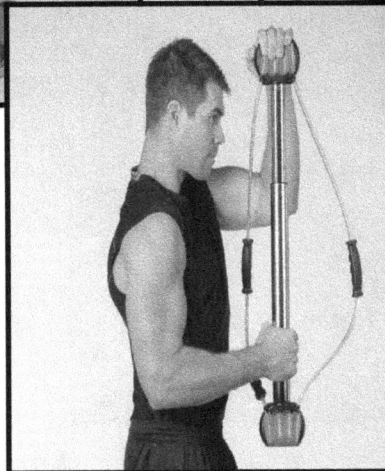

PHASE TWO

11 REP RANGE MAX X4

HOW TO PERFORM THIS ROUTINE:
REP RANGE MAX X4

Day 1=12 reps, Day 2=20 reps, Day 3=12 reps, Day 4=20 reps, Day 5=7 reps
Day 6=10 reps, Day 7=20 reps. On the last rep perform a 20 second
Isometric contraction. Perform all exercises without rest for 2 rounds.
Alternate day 1 and day 2.....7 days per week for 2 weeks

DAY ONE

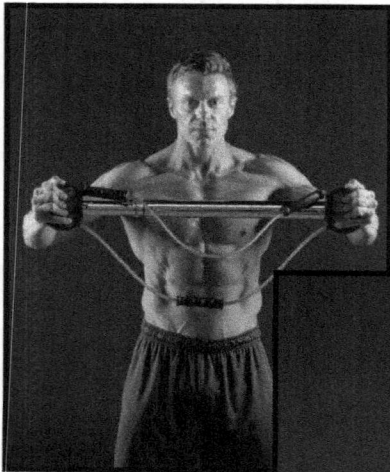

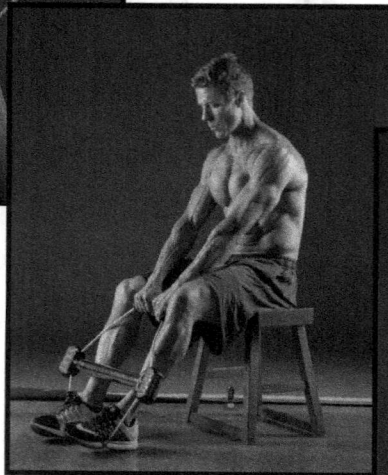

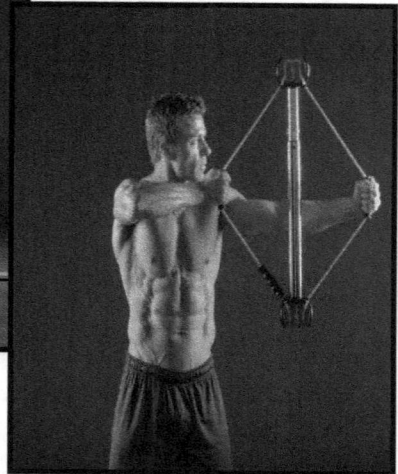

PHASE TWO

11 REP RANGE MAX X4

HOW TO PERFORM THIS ROUTINE:
REP RANGE MAX X4

Day 1=12 reps, Day 2=20 reps, Day 3=12 reps, Day 4=20 reps, Day 5=7 reps
Day 6=10 reps, Day 7=20 reps. On the last rep perform a 20 second
Isometric contraction. Perform all exercises without rest for 2 rounds.
Alternate day 1 and day 2.....7 days per week for 2 weeks

DAY ONE continued..........

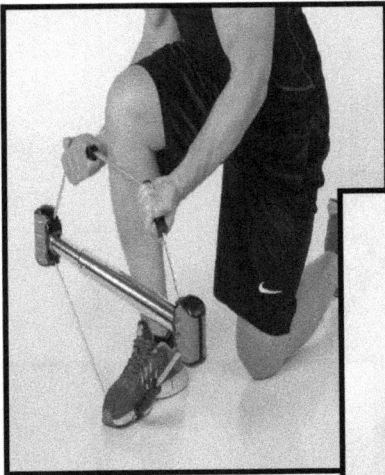

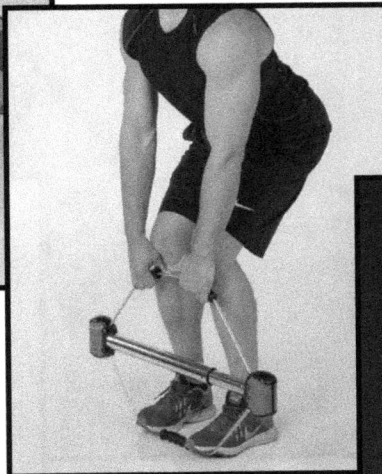

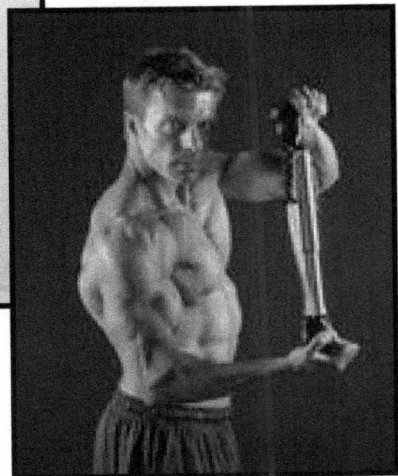

PHASE TWO

11 REP RANGE MAX X4

HOW TO PERFORM THIS ROUTINE:
REP RANGE MAX X4

Day 1=12 reps, Day 2=20 reps, Day 3=12 reps, Day 4=20 reps, Day 5=7 reps
Day 6=10 reps, Day 7=20 reps. On the last rep perform a 20 second
Isometric contraction. Perform all exercises without rest for 2 rounds.
Alternate day 1 and day 2.....7 days per week for 2 weeks

DAY ONE contin........

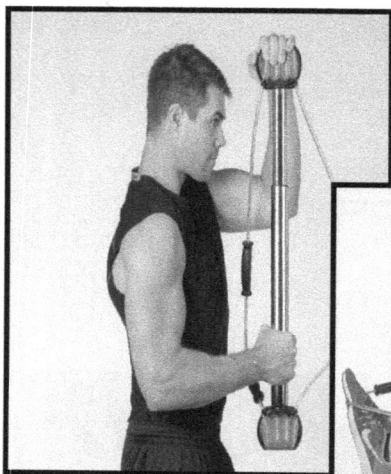

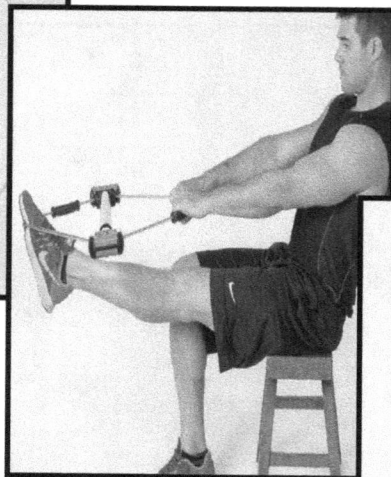

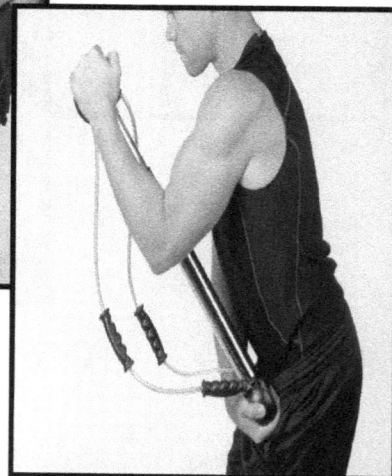

PHASE TWO

11 REP RANGE MAX X4

HOW TO PERFORM THIS ROUTINE:
REP RANGE MAX X4

Day 1=12 reps, Day 2=20 reps, Day 3=12 reps, Day 4=20 reps, Day 5=7 reps
Day 6=10 reps, Day 7=20 reps. On the last rep perform a 20 second
Isometric contraction. Perform all exercises without rest for 2 rounds.
Alternate day 1 and day 2.....7 days per week for 2 weeks

DAY TWO

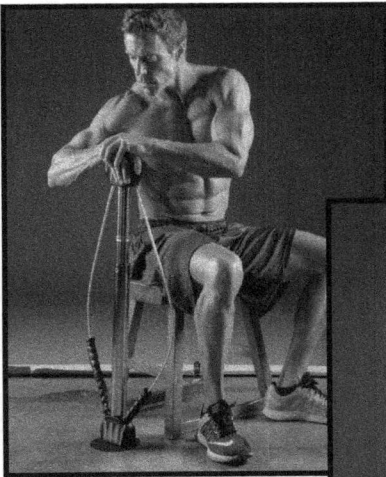
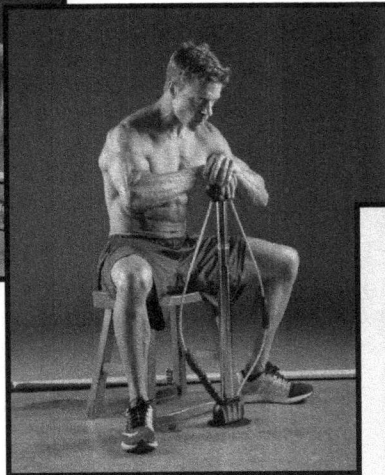
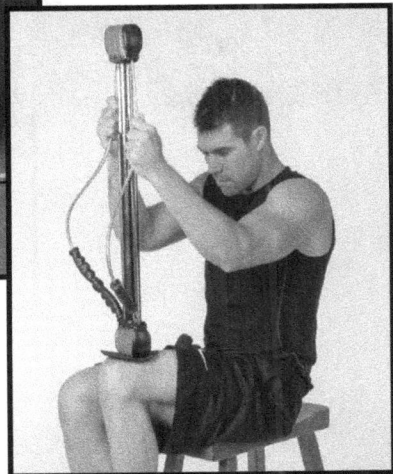

PHASE TWO

11 REP RANGE MAX X4

HOW TO PERFORM THIS ROUTINE:
REP RANGE MAX X4

Day 1=12 reps, Day 2=20 reps, Day 3=12 reps, Day 4=20 reps, Day 5=7 reps
Day 6=10 reps, Day 7=20 reps. On the last rep perform a 20 second
Isometric contraction. Perform all exercises without rest for 2 rounds.
Alternate day 1 and day 2.....7 days per week for 2 weeks

DAY TWO continued...........

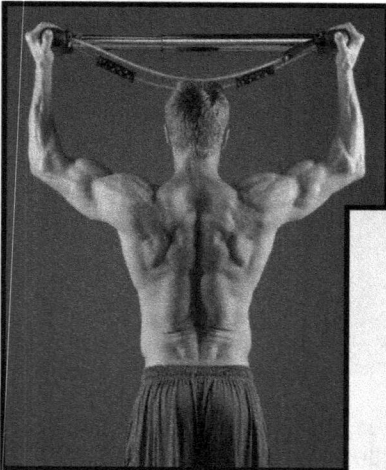
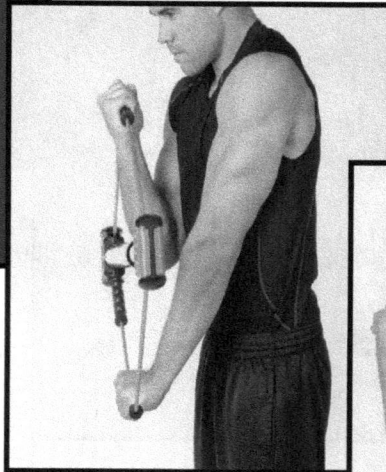
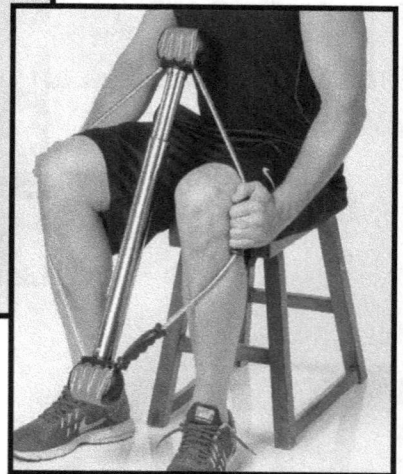

PHASE TWO

11 REP RANGE MAX X4

HOW TO PERFORM THIS ROUTINE:
REP RANGE MAX X4

Day 1=12 reps, Day 2=20 reps, Day 3=12 reps, Day 4=20 reps, Day 5=7 reps
Day 6=10 reps, Day 7=20 reps. On the last rep perform a 20 second
Isometric contraction. Perform all exercises without rest for 2 rounds.
Alternate day 1 and day 2.....7 days per week for 2 weeks

DAY TWO continued...........

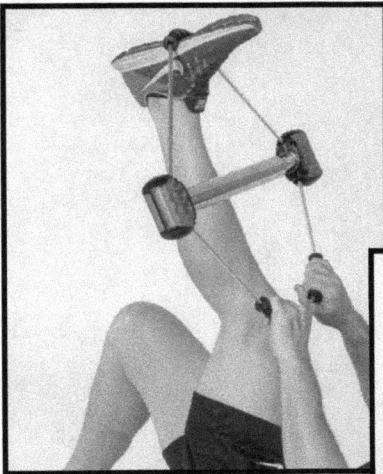

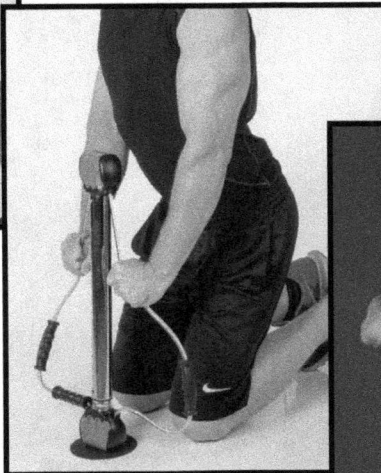

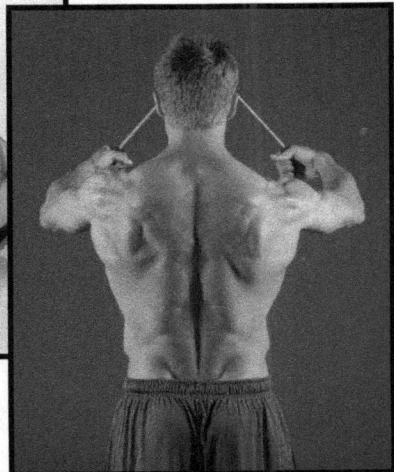

Looking forward to hearing from you on your progress. Please drop me an email skippymarl@icloud.com

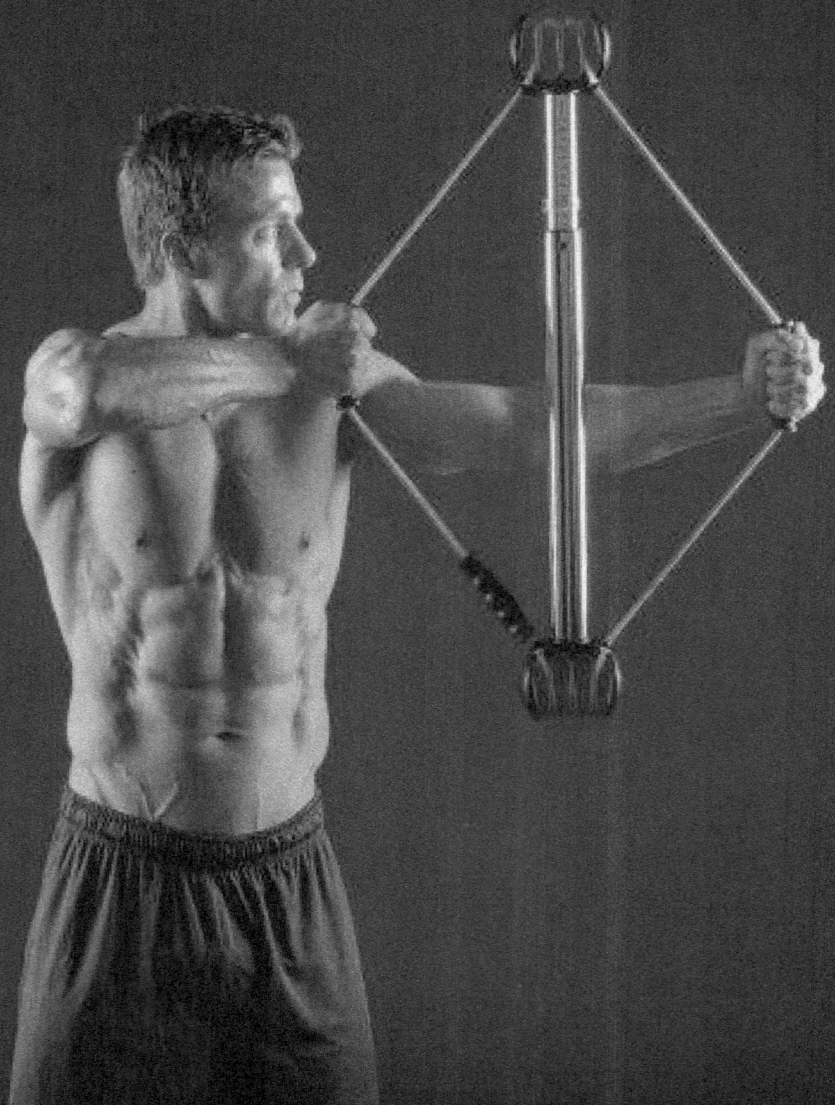

MOST IMPROVED STUDENT AWARD
COMING SOON
SEPTEMBER 31ST 2020